Explainable Machine Intelligence in Healthcare

Riccardo Ortale • Giovanni Costa •
Agostino Forestiero
Editors

Explainable Machine Intelligence in Healthcare

Springer

Editors
Riccardo Ortale
ICAR-CNR
Rende (CS), Italy

Giovanni Costa
ICAR-CNR
Rende (CS), Italy

Agostino Forestiero
ICAR-CNR
Rende (CS), Italy

ISBN 978-3-031-91378-5 ISBN 978-3-031-91379-2 (eBook)
https://doi.org/10.1007/978-3-031-91379-2

This Springer imprint is published by the registered company Springer Nature Switzerland AG
The registered company address is: Gewerbestrasse 11, 6330 Cham, Switzerland

Preface

The healthcare industry is experiencing a significant transformation driven by relentless technological advancements. Machine Intelligence (MI) is increasingly being integrated into healthcare for various tasks, including decision-making, diagnosis, treatment planning, and optimization of administrative workflows. However, a critical barrier hinders the full realization of this potential: the black-box nature of healthcare MI systems. This opacity raises concerns regarding their effectiveness, safety, privacy, accountability, and bias, eroding trust among patients, healthcare professionals, and society. Ethical considerations also come into play, as opaque healthcare MI decisions can lead to unintended consequences.

Explainable MI (XMI) is a fundamental tool that demystifies the decision-making process of MI systems in their application domains. In particular, in the healthcare domain, XMI enhances the trustworthiness of MI systems and instills confidence in stakeholders regarding their responsible contribution to healthcare decision support.

Explainable Machine Intelligence in Healthcare investigates the role of XMI in enhancing the trustworthiness of healthcare MI, thus fostering the trust of all parties involved, including patients, healthcare professionals, stakeholders, and society. It comprehensively examines XMI within healthcare, covering its foundations, opportunities, and limitations. The book showcases cutting-edge solutions, practical applications, and case studies. It also explores future directions in this rapidly evolving field, outlining possibilities for innovative research and applications.

Content of the Book

Organized into three major parts, the book delves into the fundamentals, techniques, and applications of XMI in various medical fields. This organization provides a clear and logical progression for readers, highlighting the thematic connections between chapters and facilitating a deeper understanding. In particular,

- **Part I: Fundamentals** lays the groundwork for understanding the role of XMI in healthcare. Chapter 1 titled "Supporting Healthcare Decision-Making: A Journey Through CDSS, Explainability, and Bias Mitigation with Explainable AI" analyzes the transformative role of XMI, starting with an examination of its significance and then delving into its practical applications within Clinical Decision Support Systems (CDSS). It further addresses ethical considerations and how XMI allows patients to make informed decisions aligned with their values and preferences. Chapter 2 titled "Transparent Models in Healthcare: Enhancing Decision Support Through Explainability" introduces a framework utilizing Soft Decision Trees to create inherently explainable machine learning models for medical diagnostics. These models provide global explanations without needing post-hoc methods, aiming to improve trust and cooperation in healthcare decision-making through intuitive and transparent predictions. Chapter 3 titled "Improving Explanation Measures Inside the Decision-Making Process to Increase the Potential of AI Applications in Healthcare" delves into lowering bias and strengthening the patient-physician relationship to restore trust in healthcare MI. Chapter 4 titled "Shedding Light Inside the Black Box: Techniques for Explainable Artificial Intelligence in Healthcare" provides an overview of cutting-edge XMI techniques to improve trust, help clinicians understand and contextualize MI outcomes, and ultimately enhance patient care. It also highlights that combining Large Language Models with XMI techniques can improve model interpretability, enhancing the interaction between the MI system and healthcare professionals.
- **Part II: Techniques and Methodologies** offers readers a comprehensive understanding of the latest advancements in XMI within the healthcare sector. Chapter 5 titled "Batch Integrated Gradients: A Library for Explaining Temporal Health Data" introduces a specific library for temporal explanations. Chapter 6 titled "Decision Tree Models to Select High-Risk Patients for Lung Cancer Screening and Model Interpretability" explores interpretable and post hoc explainable approaches for lung cancer screening. Chapter 7 titled "LIME and GraphLIME Coupled with a Features-Attention Mechanism for Thoracic Diagnosis Improvement" offers a discussion about the coupling of LIME and GraphLIME with a features-attention mechanism for thoracic diagnosis improvement, showcasing the practical application of these methodologies. Chapter 8 titled "Explainable Artificial Intelligence for Parkinson's Disease" offers a comprehensive and critical overview of the cutting-edge progress in XMI solutions tailored for Parkinson's disease. It focuses on the benefits, drawbacks, and clinical suitability of various XMI techniques. It also provides an in-depth review of the datasets used, the empirical findings, the significant challenges encountered, and possible solutions.
- **Part III: Case Studies and Applications** showcases the practical application of XMI in diverse medical domains through specific case studies. Chapter 9 titled "Interpreting Convolutional Neural Networks for Brain Tumors: A Transparent Box Approach" focuses on saliency maps to explore the workings of a multiclass CNN model for brain tumor classification. Chapter 10 titled "Evaluation of

Explainability Methods in Medical Image Analysis" reviews the challenges and various algorithms developed to evaluate MI decision explanations quantitatively. It emphasizes the importance of meaningful evaluations, considering the subjective nature and experience-based variability of medical decisions. Chapter 11 titled "Medical Images Analysis through Artificial Intelligence Techniques with Explainable Features" presents an advanced diagnostic framework that combines the U-Net neural network architecture with XMI techniques for analyzing chest radiographs.

Book Readership

Designed to serve as a leading reference, *Explainable Machine Intelligence in Healthcare* caters to a diverse readership.

- Academicians, researchers, and scholars will find a wealth of the latest discoveries and advanced methods for reliable analysis and diagnosis.
- Practitioners, students, and industry professionals will acquire valuable insights into the design, development, integration, and deployment of XMI in healthcare.
- Public health agencies and NGOs can utilize this knowledge to develop XMI solutions that improve public health outcomes.

Purpose and Scope

Explainable Machine Intelligence in Healthcare aims to contribute to the ongoing dialogue and development in the field of XMI in healthcare by fostering further research and innovation to enhance the trustworthiness and effectiveness of MI systems in healthcare, instill trust in stakeholders, and ultimately improve patient care and healthcare outcomes.

Rende (CS), Italy

Riccardo Ortale
Giovanni Costa
Agostino Forestiero

Acknowledgments We would like to express our gratitude to all the authors for their invaluable contributions to this book.

Contents

Part I
Fundamentals

Supporting Healthcare Decision-Making: A Journey Through CDSS, Explainability, and Bias Mitigation with Explainable AI

Mozhgan Salimiparsa, Daniel Lizotte, and Kamran Sedig

Contents

Abstract In the dynamic realm of healthcare, explainable AI (XAI) has emerged as a pivotal player in forming informed decision-making and patient-centered care. This chapter embarks on an exploration of the impact that XAI has on healthcare,

---

M. Salimiparsa (✉) · D. Lizotte · K. Sedig
Western University, London, ON, Canada
e-mail: msalimip@uwo.ca

R. Ortale et al. (eds.), *Explainable Machine Intelligence in Healthcare*,
https://doi.org/10.1007/978-3-031-91379-2_1

starting with an examination of its significance and then delving into its practical applications within Clinical Decision Support Systems (CDSS). The discussion also encompasses ethical considerations and how XAI empowers patients. At the core of this discussion lies the significance of XAI in clarifying the often opaque algorithms governing healthcare processes. In an era where trust and transparency are paramount, XAI serves as a guiding light, providing healthcare professionals with insights into the decision-making processes of AI-driven systems. By explaining the rationale behind AI-generated recommendations, XAI cultivates trust and confidence in these technologies, ultimately enhancing the quality and safety of patient care. Furthermore, we delve into the practical applications of XAI within CDSS, where it enhances the capabilities of healthcare providers by enabling more informed and precise clinical decisions. Through real-world examples, we observe the tangible benefits of integrating XAI into healthcare delivery. However, our exploration does not end with technical advancements; it extends into the realm of ethical considerations. We pause to reflect on the ethical implications of deploying AI in healthcare, addressing concerns such as accountability, bias mitigation, and the protection of patient rights. Amid these complexities, there emerges a promising outcome—the empowerment of patients. Transparent and interpretable AI models enable patients to play an active role in their healthcare journey. Equipped with a deeper understanding of their health conditions and treatment options, patients are empowered to make informed decisions aligned with their values and preferences. On this journey through the realm of XAI in healthcare, our goal is to provide readers with a comprehensive understanding of its transformative potential and profound implications. By the end of this chapter, we hope readers will not only grasp the complexities of XAI but also envision a future where technology serves as a facilitator of positive transformations in healthcare, promoting effectiveness, efficiency, ethics, and equity.

Keywords Explainable AI (XAI) · Clinical Decision Support Systems (CDSS) · Healthcare decision-making · Patient-centered care · AI transparency · AI ethics · Bias mitigation in AI · AI in healthcare · Patient empowerment · AI explainability

1 Overview of Explainable AI in Healthcare

1.1 Introduction

In recent years, artificial intelligence (AI) has emerged as a transformative force in the field of healthcare, revolutionizing the way medical professionals diagnose, treat, and monitor patients [1]. Leveraging advanced algorithms and vast datasets, AI systems have demonstrated remarkable capabilities in tasks ranging from medical imaging analysis to drug discovery. The applications of AI in healthcare are vast and diverse, encompassing various facets of medical practice. AI-powered systems are utilized for diagnosing diseases, planning treatment strategies, monitoring patient vital signs, and personalizing medicine regimens. For instance, machine learning algorithms can analyze medical images such as X-rays and MRIs to detect anomalies and assist radiologists in making accurate diagnoses [2]. Additionally, AI-driven predictive analytics models enable healthcare providers to identify patients at risk of developing certain conditions, allowing for proactive interventions and improved outcomes [3]. As the adoption of AI continues to rise, there is a growing recognition of the need for transparency and interpretability in healthcare AI applications [4, 5].

1.2 The Need for Explainability in Healthcare AI

While AI holds great promise for enhancing healthcare delivery, the lack of transparency and interpretability in AI models poses significant challenges [6]. Given the life-or-death consequences of healthcare decisions, it is imperative that AI models are transparent and interpretable to both healthcare professionals and patients. Opaque AI systems, often referred to as "black box" models, hinder clinicians' ability to understand the reasoning behind AI-generated recommendations or predictions. This opacity can lead to distrust among healthcare professionals and patients, raising concerns about bias, fairness, and potential medical errors [7, 8]. Explainable AI (XAI) emerges as a critical solution to address these challenges by providing insights into how AI models arrive at their conclusions. By making AI algorithms more transparent and interpretable, XAI facilitates collaboration between AI systems and human stakeholders.

1.3 What Is Explainable AI (XAI)

Explainable AI (XAI) refers to a set of techniques and methodologies designed to enhance the transparency and interpretability of AI models [9]. Unlike traditional black box AI models, which operate as inscrutable entities, explainable AI models offer insights into their inner workings, making their decisions more understandable to human users. XAI techniques encompass a variety of approaches, including rule-based systems, model-agnostic methods, and interpretable machine learning algorithms.

For example, rule-based systems employ a set of predefined rules to make decisions, allowing clinicians to understand the logic behind each recommendation [10]. Model-agnostic methods, such as LIME (local interpretable model-agnostic explanations), generate explanations for AI predictions by perturbing input features and observing changes in model outputs [11]. Interpretable machine learning algorithms, such as decision trees and linear models, produce transparent representations of learned patterns, enabling users to interpret model predictions with ease [12].

1.4 Benefits of Explainable AI in Healthcare

The integration of explainable AI into healthcare offers numerous benefits for patients, clinicians, and regulatory authorities alike. By enhancing the interpretability of AI models, XAI has the potential to facilitate clinical decision-making, enabling healthcare providers to validate AI-generated recommendations and understand the rationale behind treatment plans [13]. Moreover, explainable AI can contribute to improve patient outcomes by promoting transparency and engagement in the healthcare process [14].

Furthermore, XAI plays a crucial role in ensuring regulatory compliance and addressing ethical considerations in healthcare AI applications [15]. By providing transparency into AI systems' decision-making processes, XAI helps mitigate the risks of bias, discrimination, and unintended consequences, thereby safeguarding patient safety and privacy [16].

1.5 Challenges and Limitations of XAI in Healthcare

Despite its potential benefits, the implementation of explainable AI in healthcare is not without challenges. One of the primary obstacles is the complexity of healthcare data, which often consists of heterogeneous sources, incomplete records, and noisy information. This data complexity poses challenges for interpretable model development and may require sophisticated feature engineering techniques to extract meaningful insights.

Additionally, achieving model interpretability while maintaining high predictive performance remains a significant challenge in XAI research. Many existing interpretable machine learning algorithms sacrifice predictive accuracy for transparency [17], limiting their practical utility in real-world healthcare settings. Balancing the trade-off between interpretability and performance is an ongoing area of research in XAI [18–20], with researchers exploring novel techniques to reconcile these competing objectives.

1.6 Future Directions and Emerging Trends

Looking ahead, the future of explainable AI in healthcare is ripe with opportunities for innovation and advancement. Emerging trends in XAI research aim to address existing limitations and push the boundaries of interpretability in AI models.

One key direction is the integration of domain knowledge and expert insights into XAI models. While AI algorithms excel at analyzing large volumes of data and identifying patterns, they may lack the contextual understanding and domain-specific knowledge possessed by human experts. By incorporating domain knowledge into

XAI models, researchers can improve the relevance and accuracy of the explanations provided by these models. This approach leverages expert knowledge to guide the interpretation process and ensure that the explanations generated by AI systems are clinically relevant and actionable.

Additionally, there is growing interest in developing interactive XAI tools that enable users to explore and interact with AI models in real time. Traditional XAI techniques typically provide static explanations that offer limited insights into the underlying decision-making process. Interactive XAI tools, on the other hand, empower users to probe AI models, ask questions, and receive immediate feedback. These tools can facilitate collaboration between healthcare professionals and AI systems, enabling more informed decision-making and fostering transparency in AI-driven healthcare applications.

Furthermore, there is a need to develop standardized evaluation metrics and benchmarks for assessing the performance of XAI models in healthcare settings. Currently, there is a lack of consensus on how to measure the interpretability of AI systems, making it challenging to compare and evaluate different XAI techniques. By establishing standardized evaluation frameworks, researchers can ensure the reproducibility and generalizability of XAI research and facilitate the adoption of interpretable AI models in clinical practice.

Overall, the future of XAI in healthcare is characterized by a diverse range of opportunities and challenges. By embracing emerging trends and advancing research in XAI, we can unlock the full potential of AI technologies to improve patient outcomes, enhance clinical decision-making, and transform healthcare delivery.

2 Applications of XAI in Clinical Decision Support

2.1 Introduction

Clinical Decision Support Systems (CDSS) leverage computational algorithms to provide actionable insights and recommendations, aiding clinicians in making informed decisions regarding patient care. By leveraging AI and machine learning techniques, CDSS can sift through immense amounts of data to identify patterns, trends, and potential risks that may go unnoticed by human clinicians. This ability to process and analyze complex datasets makes CDSS invaluable in diagnosing diseases, predicting treatment outcomes, and optimizing patient care pathways.

However, the increasing adoption of AI and machine learning algorithms in CDSS has raised concerns regarding the opacity of these systems. Traditional black box AI models, while often effective in generating accurate predictions, lack transparency and interpretability, posing significant challenges in the context of healthcare [21]. In response to these challenges, explainable artificial intelligence (XAI) has emerged as a critical paradigm shift in the field of healthcare AI. XAI aims to provide transparent and interpretable outputs from AI models, enabling clinicians to understand the rationale behind CDSS recommendations and make informed decisions regarding patient care.

2.2 The Need for XAI in CDSS

Traditional black box AI models, characterized by their complex and opaque decision-making processes, are ill-suited for healthcare applications. In the context of CDSS, where decisions directly impact patient outcomes, the lack of transparency in AI algorithms poses significant risks. Clinicians are understandably hesitant to rely on recommendations from AI systems that they cannot understand or trust.

Moreover, ethical, legal, and regulatory frameworks mandate transparency and interpretability in healthcare AI systems [22]. Patients have the right to understand the basis of decisions affecting their care, and clinicians must be able to justify and explain recommendations provided by CDSS. Failure to meet these requirements not only compromises patient safety but also exposes healthcare providers to legal and regulatory scrutiny.

2.3 Integration of XAI into CDSS

Integrating XAI techniques into existing CDSS frameworks presents both opportunities and challenges. On one hand, XAI has the potential to enhance the transparency and interpretability of AI-driven recommendations, thereby increasing clinician adoption. On the other hand, implementing XAI in real-world healthcare settings requires careful consideration of various factors, including technical feasibility, scalability, and usability.

One of the primary opportunities afforded by integrating XAI into CDSS is the ability to provide clinicians with transparent explanations for AI-driven recommendations. Many CDSS rely on complex machine learning algorithms to analyze patient data and provide treatment suggestions. However, these algorithms often operate as "black boxes," making it challenging for clinicians to understand the underlying reasoning behind their recommendations. By incorporating XAI methods, CDSS can generate interpretable explanations for their predictions, enabling clinicians to better understand the recommendations provided. Furthermore, integrating XAI into CDSS can help address concerns related to algorithmic bias and fairness. AI algorithms trained on biased data may inadvertently perpetuate disparities in healthcare delivery, leading to inequitable treatment outcomes. XAI techniques can facilitate the identification and mitigation of biases in CDSS by providing insights into the factors driving algorithmic decisions. Clinicians can use these explanations to assess the fairness and reliability of AI-driven recommendations and take appropriate action to address any disparities.

However, the integration of XAI into CDSS also poses several challenges. One major consideration is the technical feasibility, as many XAI techniques rely on access to detailed patient data and advanced computational resources. This means ensuring that the necessary infrastructure and data resources are in place to support the implementation of XAI within CDSS. Additionally, the integration of XAI may raise concerns about data security, as the handling of sensitive patient information must adhere to strict privacy regulations and security protocols to safeguard patient confidentiality and prevent unauthorized access.

Additionally, scalability is a key concern for both CDSS and XAI. CDSS must be able to handle the diverse needs of various healthcare organizations and cope with the increasing volume of patient data generated in clinical settings. Similarly, XAI techniques need to be scalable to provide explanations effectively, especially as the complexity and size of the data being analyzed continue to grow. Ensuring scalability for both CDSS and XAI is essential for the successful integration of explainable AI into healthcare systems.

Moreover, the usability of XAI-enabled CDSS is critical to their successful adoption by healthcare professionals. Clinicians are often pressed for time and may be resistant to adopting new technologies that disrupt their established workflows. Therefore, XAI solutions must be designed with the end user in mind, providing intuitive interfaces and actionable insights that enhance, rather than hinder, clinical decision-making.

In summary, while integrating XAI into CDSS offers significant benefits in terms of transparency, fairness, and trustworthiness, it also presents challenges related to technical feasibility, scalability, and usability. By addressing these challenges and leveraging the opportunities afforded by XAI, healthcare organizations can develop more effective and equitable decision support systems that improve patient outcomes and enhance the quality of care.

2.4 *Case Studies and Examples*

In recent years, there has been a growing body of academic research focused on integrating XAI methodologies into CDSS to enhance interpretability and transparency of these systems within the healthcare sector. In this section, we explore several case studies and applications of XAI in CDSS across different medical specialties.

Amoroso et al. [23] investigated the application of an XAI framework in the context of breast cancer therapies. They employed clustering and dimension reduction methods to outline significant clinical features for oncological patients' profiling. Their experiments showcased the effectiveness of this method not just in identifying essential clinical features but also in defining the patient's profile, specifically assigning them to the relevant cluster. Nagaraj et al. [24] utilized XAI methods to assist in attribute selection, integration, prediction, and rule mining for a diabetic organization. This study proposes a method for diabetes prediction and a recommendation system. Various machine learning algorithms including XGBoost, support vector machine (SVM), random forest classifier, and decision tree are employed to build the prediction model. The best-performing algorithm is selected for optimal accuracy. The LIME explainer is then utilized to assess the accuracy of diabetic positive and negative patients in a tabular format.

El-Sappagh et al. [25] introduced a random forest (RF) model designed for diagnosing Alzheimer's disease (AD) and detecting its progression. Utilizing SHAP, they provided detailed explanations for individual patient diagnoses or predictions of progression, highlighting the impacts of various features. Additionally, they employed a fuzzy rule-based system to generate natural language interpretations, aiding patients and physicians in understanding the AI model. This proposed system aims to improve clinical understanding of AD diagnosis and progression by offering insights into how different factors influence disease risk. Shad et al. [26] aimed to leverage neural network models and a hybrid dataset to detect Alzheimer's disease early on. It employed a hybrid dataset and studied four separate classifications. The paper explored the exact regions associated with each specific classification for the patients and utilized the LIME-based XAI framework to explain the models' decisions.

Kavya et al. [27] proposed a computer-aided framework for allergy diagnoses, leveraging multiple machine learning (ML) algorithms. To ensure interpretability, they adopted a rule-based approach using a random forest model. Each decision path in the tree was transformed into IF-THEN rules, providing transparent explanations derived from medical data. Wu et al. [28] proposed a novel method called counterfactual multi-granularity graph supporting fact extraction (CMGE) for diagnosing lymphedema. This graph extracts factual information from electronic medical records (EMRs) and has the capability to discern causal relationships between features and diagnostic outcomes through counterfactual intervention. Experimental findings from real Chinese electronic medical records on lymphedema not only confirm the accuracy of the approach for diagnoses but also demonstrate its ability to provide precise supporting evidence for the results.

It is important to note that the case studies presented in this section represent only a subset of the broader landscape of applications for XAI in CDSS. For those seeking a more comprehensive understanding, there are several surveys available [21, 29] that specifically review the application of XAI in CDSS, providing additional insights and perspectives.

2.5 Future Directions and Challenges

As XAI continues to evolve, future advancements hold the promise of further enhancing the transparency, interpretability, and trustworthiness of CDSS in healthcare. However, several challenges must be addressed to realize the full potential of XAI in clinical practice. Scalability, robustness, and generalizability remain ongoing concerns, requiring continued research and innovation to overcome.

Additionally, as healthcare AI systems become increasingly integrated into clinical workflows, ethical and societal implications must be carefully considered. Ensuring fairness, accountability, and transparency in AI-driven decision-making processes is essential to maintaining patient trust and confidence in CDSS.

In conclusion, the integration of XAI into CDSS represents a significant step forward in the quest for transparent, interpretable, and trustworthy healthcare AI systems. By enabling clinicians to understand and trust the recommendations provided by AI models, XAI has the potential to revolutionize clinical decision-making processes and improve patient outcomes in healthcare. However, realizing this potential requires collaboration across disciplines and continued investment in research, development, and implementation efforts.

3 Ethical Considerations in Explainable AI for Healthcare

3.1 Introduction

In recent years, the integration of artificial intelligence (AI) in healthcare has rapidly advanced, offering promising solutions to improve patient outcomes and streamline medical processes. However, along with these advancements come ethical challenges that must be carefully navigated to ensure the responsible and ethical deployment of AI technologies in healthcare settings. This section of the chapter explores the ethical considerations surrounding explainable AI (XAI) in healthcare, focusing on issues such as patient privacy, transparency, algorithm bias, fairness, and regulatory compliance, and then we talk about the future directions of XAI in this regard.

3.2 Ethical Challenges in Healthcare AI

The integration of AI and machine learning (ML) in healthcare, while promising substantial improvements, raises various ethical challenges that need to be carefully considered to ensure responsible and equitable use of these technologies [30].

One of the primary ethical considerations is the need for transparency and accountability in AI-driven decision-making processes. Traditional black box AI models, which operate without providing insights into their inner workings, raise concerns about the potential for bias, discrimination, and lack of accountability. Explainable AI (XAI) techniques aim to address these concerns by providing interpretable explanations for AI predictions and recommendations. By making the decision-making process transparent and understandable to healthcare professionals and patients, XAI enhances accountability and facilitates trust in AI systems.

Moreover, XAI plays a crucial role in ensuring the fairness and equity of AI-driven healthcare applications. Bias in AI algorithms, whether due to skewed training data or inherent algorithmic biases, can lead to disparities in healthcare outcomes among different demographic groups. For example, a predictive model for disease diagnosis trained on biased data may systematically underdiagnose certain demographic groups, leading to unequal access to care and treatment. XAI techniques enable the identification and mitigation of bias by providing insights into the factors influencing AI predictions. By detecting and correcting bias in AI models, XAI helps to promote fairness and ensure that healthcare resources are distributed equitably across diverse patient populations. This is particularly important in addressing ethical concerns in healthcare, such as informed consent, patient autonomy, privacy, fairness, and nondiscrimination. Here's how XAI can help in addressing these ethical considerations:

1. *Informed Consent and Patient Autonomy*: Informed consent requires that patients are fully aware of the risks, benefits, and implications of AI-generated recommendations. XAI can enhance the process of obtaining informed consent by making the functionalities and decision-making processes of AI systems transparent. Patients can make better-informed decisions about their care when they understand how medical recommendations are derived from AI systems. This clarity supports the ethical principle of respect for persons and autonomy, ensuring that patients' consent is truly informed [31].
2. *Privacy and Data Protection*: XAI can play a role in safeguarding privacy and ensuring the ethical use of patient data. By making the data processing mechanisms of AI systems transparent, XAI can help in ensuring that data use complies with legal and ethical standards, reducing the risk of unauthorized data exploitation or breaches [32].
3. *Fairness and Nondiscrimination*: Explainability in AI helps to identify and mitigate biases in AI algorithms, promoting fairness and preventing discrimination in healthcare services. XAI enables stakeholders to examine and correct biases in AI systems, ensuring equitable and ethical treatment of all patients regardless of their background [33–35].
4. *Ethical Compliance and Transparency*: XAI fosters ethical compliance by making AI systems more transparent and understandable, which is crucial for healthcare providers and patients to trust and reliably use AI-based medical services [15]. Transparent AI systems can demonstrate their adherence to ethical norms and regulations, facilitating ethical audits and accountability.

3.3 Artificial Intelligence (AI) and Algorithmic Bias in Healthcare

AI can perpetuate biases inherent in the data it is trained on, while also serving as a tool for identifying and mitigating these biases. When AI algorithms learn from biased data—stemming from historical inequalities or skewed sampling—they risk amplifying these biases in their decisions [36]. This phenomenon is observed across various sectors, including healthcare, criminal justice, and financial services, where AI-driven decisions profoundly impact human lives.

For example, in healthcare, AI systems used for diagnosing diseases or predicting patient outcomes may inadvertently perpetuate biases if they are trained on datasets lacking diversity. This can lead to disparities in healthcare outcomes, such as misdiagnoses or delayed treatment for patients from underrepresented groups. To address these challenges, explainable AI (XAI) techniques can be employed to provide insights into the decision-making processes of AI models. XAI allows healthcare professionals to understand how AI arrives at its decisions, facilitating the identification and correction of biases.

Furthermore, XAI can aid in the development of fairer algorithms by analyzing datasets for patterns of bias and designing models that explicitly account for and correct these biases. By integrating XAI into healthcare AI systems, stakeholders can ensure transparency and fairness in decision-making processes, ultimately leading to more accurate diagnoses and equitable treatment options for diverse patient populations.

The concept of explainability in AI models is crucial in this context, serving as an essential mechanism for developers and clinicians to uncover and address biases. During the initial phases of AI model development and validation, it is optimal to scrutinize and mitigate bias through processes that involve identifying and adjusting critical features that may indicate bias. Additionally, there is a moral obligation to reduce AI bias, not only to improve model accuracy and fairness but also to meet ethical standards. This necessitates the proactive involvement of developers and clinicians in identifying and mitigating potential imperfections and limitations of AI applications, particularly the risk of misallocating resources and engaging in discriminatory practices due to biased AI constructs. Therefore, explainability is not merely a technical aspect but also an ethical imperative to ensure fairness in the application of AI in medicine.

3.4 Approaches for Bias Assessment and Mitigation

XAI offers a promising avenue for addressing bias in AI systems by providing transparency and interpretability into the decision-making processes of these systems. By elucidating how AI algorithms arrive at their conclusions, XAI enables stakeholders to identify and rectify biases effectively. Several methodologies within the realm of XAI have emerged as powerful tools for bias mitigation:

1. *Model Interpretation Techniques*: Model interpretation techniques represent a foundational pillar of XAI, offering invaluable insights into the inner workings of complex AI models. By peeling back the layers of abstraction, these techniques aim to elucidate the decision-making process, facilitating a deeper understanding

of model behavior and enabling stakeholders to pinpoint potential sources of bias. One such technique is feature importance analysis, which quantifies the contribution of each feature to the model's predictions, thereby highlighting influential factors and potential biases. Partial dependence plots provide a visual depiction of how the model's predictions change with variations in individual features, offering intuitive insights into the relationship between inputs and outputs. Additionally, local interpretable model-agnostic explanations (LIME) offer granular explanations for individual predictions, allowing stakeholders to discern the rationale behind specific model decisions. By harnessing these interpretation techniques, stakeholders gain the tools necessary to identify and address biases effectively, fostering transparency and accountability in AI systems.

2. *Fairness-Aware Learning*: Fairness-aware learning techniques represent a proactive approach to bias mitigation, integrating fairness considerations directly into the model training process [37, 38]. These techniques recognize the inherent challenges posed by biased data and aim to mitigate biases at their root, thereby promoting equity and fairness in decision-making. By incorporating fairness constraints or regularization terms into the training objective, fairness-aware learning ensures that the model's predictions are equitable across different demographic groups, guarding against discriminatory outcomes. Adversarial learning approaches, such as adversarial debiasing and adversarial training [38, 39], augment fairness-aware learning by training models to withstand adversarial attacks aimed at inducing discriminatory behavior. By exposing models to adversarial examples during training [40], these approaches bolster the model's resilience to biases, thereby enhancing the robustness and fairness of AI systems.
3. *Bias Detection and Mitigation*: XAI methodologies encompass a diverse array of techniques for detecting and mitigating bias post-model deployment. Bias detection methods serve as a critical first step, scrutinizing model predictions to identify disparities in outcomes across demographic groups [41]. These methods provide valuable insights into the presence and magnitude of biases, laying the groundwork for targeted interventions. Bias mitigation techniques then come into play, aiming to rectify these disparities and promote fairness in decision-making. Strategies such as reweighting training data and algorithmic debiasing adjust model predictions to achieve equitable outcomes, recalibrating the model's learning process to counteract the influence of biased samples [42, 43]. Moreover, counterfactual interpretation offers a nuanced approach to bias mitigation, involving the systematic manipulation of input data to observe changes in predictions. By perturbing input features and analyzing resulting alterations in predictions, stakeholders gain insights into potential sources of bias and devise tailored interventions to address them effectively [44, 45]. Additionally, attention mechanisms within AI models play a crucial role in bias mitigation, automatically identifying salient features in data that significantly influence decision-making processes [46]. By shedding light on the underlying factors driving predictions, attention mechanisms empower stakeholders to uncover biased or sensitive attributes, facilitating targeted interventions to mitigate their impact. Furthermore, adversarial testing emerges as a pivotal technique for

assessing and quantifying biases present within AI models. By subjecting models to tailored datasets designed to reveal and quantify existing biases, adversarial testing serves as a rigorous stress test, uncovering vulnerabilities and guiding efforts to enhance fairness and equity in AI systems [47].

Collectively, these methodologies represent a multifaceted approach to bias mitigation within AI, fostering transparency, equity, and accountability in the deployment of AI systems. By leveraging these techniques, stakeholders can navigate the complexities of bias in AI and pave the way toward a more ethical and inclusive future.

3.5 Ensuring Ethical AI Design and Deployment

Ethical AI design and deployment in healthcare demand adherence to principles of fairness, accountability, and human-centered design [48]. Human-centered design principles emphasize the importance of designing AI systems with the needs and preferences of endusers—both healthcare professionals and patients—in mind. This involves soliciting feedback from stakeholders throughout the design process, prioritizing usability and accessibility, and incorporating safeguards to protect against unintended consequences or misuse of AI technologies.

3.6 Future Directions and Challenges

The complex ethical and regulatory landscape surrounding AI in healthcare poses multifaceted challenges that require careful navigation and adherence to ethical principles and legal frameworks. Ethical considerations, such as transparency, fairness, accountability, and patient autonomy, must be integrated into the design, development, and deployment of AI systems to mitigate the risk of bias, discrimination, and unintended consequences.

As AI technologies continue to evolve and permeate various aspects of healthcare delivery, new ethical dilemmas are likely to emerge, necessitating ongoing dialogue and collaboration among stakeholders. These dilemmas may include issues related to algorithmic fairness, accountability, transparency, patient consent, and the allocation of decision-making responsibility between humans and machines. Proactive engagement in interdisciplinary discussions and the development of ethical frameworks and guidelines are essential to address these emerging challenges and ensure the responsible and equitable use of AI in healthcare.

In conclusion, addressing the ongoing challenges associated with AI in healthcare requires a multifaceted approach that encompasses technical, ethical, legal, and regulatory considerations.

By prioritizing robustness and reliability, addressing data privacy and security concerns, navigating the complex ethical and regulatory landscape, and anticipating and addressing emerging ethical dilemmas, stakeholders can foster the responsible and ethical use of AI to enhance patient care and healthcare outcomes. However, achieving this vision requires a concerted effort from all stakeholders to foster a culture of ethical awareness, responsibility, and innovation in the healthcare AI ecosystem.

4 Patient-Centered XAI Solutions

4.1 Introduction

Patient-centered care focuses on treating patients as active participants in their healthcare, respecting their individual values and needs. It advocates for shared decision-making, where patients and clinicians work together to decide on the best course of action based on the patient's unique situation. This process is facilitated by tools like conversation aids, which help guide discussions during clinical encounters by providing information on medical conditions, risks, and treatment options [49].

However, the rise of AI in healthcare, particularly the use of non-transparent, "black box" models for decision support, poses a challenge to this patient-centered approach. These models do not allow clinicians to understand or explain how decisions are made, which conflicts with the principles of shared decision-making and informed patient choice.

Explainable AI (XAI) offers a solution by making the decision-making process transparent, providing clinicians and patients with insights into how AI models arrive at their recommendations. This transparency can help in tailoring conversations to the patient's individual risk factors and preferences, thus enhancing the shared decision-making process. Explainable AI can also improve patients' understanding of their conditions and treatment options, potentially leading to better engagement in their care and decision-making processes.

4.2 Design Principles for Patient-Centered XAI Solutions

Developing patient-centered XAI solutions requires adherence to key design principles that prioritize transparency, inclusivity, and user-centeredness [50]. Involving patients in the design process from the outset ensures that AI systems are aligned with their needs and preferences. Clear communication and understandable explanations are essential for building trust and fostering collaboration between patients and healthcare providers. Additionally, designers must be mindful of the potential impact of algorithmic decisions on patient outcomes and strive to mitigate biases and disparities through thoughtful design choices.

4.3 The Role of XAI in Personalization in Healthcare

Explainability in AI-powered decision aids is integral to patient-centered care, promoting transparency and shared decision-making [51]. Employing XAI techniques allows for direct explanations to patients, empowering them to comprehend and engage with their treatment plans and healthcare decisions. Transparent and understandable AI-driven recommendations foster patient empowerment, leading to improved adherence and outcomes. For instance, in a Clinical Decision Support (CDS) system, XAI can elucidate how a treatment recommendation was derived, considering patient data, clinical guidelines, and relevant research. This transparency cultivates trust and collaboration between healthcare providers and patients, ensuring decisions align with individual needs and preferences.

Transparency is paramount in patient-centered care, ensuring patients understand the reasoning behind medical recommendations. XAI methodologies provide insight into AI algorithms' inner workings, shedding light on factors influencing outcomes. By demystifying decision-making, XAI empowers patients to actively engage in their care, fostering collaboration between healthcare providers and patients.

Moreover, XAI enhances trust in healthcare AI systems by revealing the underlying logic behind AI-driven decisions [52]. Unlike black box AI models, XAI techniques enable healthcare providers and patients to understand how algorithms arrive at conclusions, promoting trust and confidence in the technology.

Furthermore, XAI promotes fairness by identifying and mitigating biases and discrimination [7]. By providing transparency, XAI techniques allow healthcare providers to assess whether algorithms inadvertently favor certain demographic groups. This transparency facilitates the development of fairer AI models that consider diverse patient needs, irrespective of race, ethnicity, gender, or socioeconomic status.

Additionally, XAI enables personalization in healthcare by tailoring treatment recommendations based on patient-specific characteristics and preferences [53]. Interpretable explanations empower healthcare providers to understand how patient demographics, medical history, and lifestyle choices influence treatment outcomes, improving patient satisfaction, adherence, and health outcomes.

4.4 Future Directions and Implications

XAI techniques have been employed to provide explanations directly to patients, enabling them to understand and engage with their treatment plans and healthcare decisions. By making AI-driven recommendations transparent and understandable, patients are empowered to actively participate in their care, leading to improved adherence and outcomes. Looking ahead, the future of patient-centered XAI solutions holds promise for advancing healthcare delivery, patient engagement, and outcomes. Emerging trends such as personalized medicine, remote monitoring, and virtual care present new opportunities for leveraging XAI to tailor interventions to individual patient needs. However, challenges such as interoperability, scalability, and regulatory compliance must be addressed to realize the full potential of patient-centered XAI solutions. By embracing transparency, accountability, and patient empowerment, healthcare stakeholders can harness the power of AI to transform healthcare delivery and improve patient outcomes.

Despite the promising benefits of XAI in patient-centered CDS systems, challenges remain, including the complexity of generating interpretable explanations, the need for interdisciplinary collaboration between AI researchers and healthcare professionals, and the integration of XAI into existing clinical workflows. Addressing these challenges presents opportunities for further research and innovation in this field.

In conclusion, XAI serves as a cornerstone in enhancing patient-centered systems and clinical decision support platforms. By leveraging XAI methodologies, healthcare organizations can unlock the full potential of AI while prioritizing patient welfare. As the intersection of AI and healthcare evolves, the principles embodied by XAI will continue to guide the progression of healthcare provision toward a more patient-centric and equitable future.

5 Conclusion

In conclusion, this chapter has provided a comprehensive overview of explainable artificial intelligence (XAI) in healthcare, exploring its various dimensions and applications. It is evident that XAI plays a pivotal role in enhancing clinical decision support systems, promoting ethical standards, and empowering patients to make well-informed choices. The journey of incorporating XAI into healthcare decision-making, with its focus on transparency, explainability, and bias mitigation, holds significant promise for reshaping and enhancing the healthcare landscape.

Reflecting on the potential of XAI, it is apparent that its adoption signifies a meaningful progression toward a future where technology not only supports clinical practices but also ensures healthcare delivery is marked by integrity, fairness, and patient-centricity.

As we continue to advance the field of XAI in healthcare, it is imperative to remain vigilant about the ethical implications and strive for inclusive and patient-centric solutions. By embracing the principles of transparency, accountability, and fairness, we can navigate the complexities of XAI implementation and pave the way for a healthcare ecosystem that prioritizes the well-being and autonomy of patients while leveraging the potential of cutting-edge technology.

References

1. Harry A. The future of medicine: harnessing the power of AI for revolutionizing healthcare. Int J Multidiscip Sci Arts. 2023;2(1):36–47.
2. Siddiq M. Ml-based medical image analysis for anomaly detection in CT scans, x-rays, and MRIs. Devot J Res Commun Serv. 2020;2(1):53–64.
3. Billings J, Dixon J, Mijanovich T, Wennberg D. Case finding for patients at risk of readmission to hospital: development of algorithm to identify high risk patients. BMJ. 2006;333(7563):327.
4. Vellido A. The importance of interpretability and visualization in machine learning for applications in medicine and health care. Neural Comput & Applic. 2020;32(24):18069–83.
5. Kiseleva A, Kotzinos D, De Hert P. Transparency of AI in healthcare as a multilayered system of accountabilities: between legal requirements and technical limitations. Front Artif Intell. 2022;5:879603.
6. Vyas B. Explainable AI: assessing methods to make AI systems more transparent and interpretable. Int J New Media Stud Int Peer Rev Sch Index J. 2023;10(1):236–42.
7. Ueda D, Kakinuma T, Fujita S, Kamagata K, Fushimi Y, Ito R, et al. Fairness of artificial intelligence in healthcare: review and recommendations. Jpn J Radiol. 2024;42(1):3–15.
8. Durán JM, Jongsma KR. Who is afraid of black box algorithms? On the epistemological and ethical basis of trust in medical AI. J Med Ethics. 2021;47(5):329–35.
9. Arrieta AB, Díaz-Rodríguez N, Del Ser J, Bennetot A, Tabik S, Barbado A, et al. Explainable artificial intelligence (XAI): concepts, taxonomies, opportunities and challenges toward responsible AI. Inf Fusion. 2020;58:82–115.
10. Macha D, Kozielski M, Wróbel Ł, Sikora M. RuleXAI – a package for rule-based explanations of machine learning model. SoftwareX. 2022;20:101209.
11. Ribeiro MT, Singh S, Guestrin C. "Why should i trust you?" Explaining the predictions of any classifier. In: Proceedings of the 22nd ACM SIGKDD international conference on knowledge discovery and data mining; 2016. p. 1135–44.
12. Molnar C. Interpretable machine learning. Lulu. com; 2020.
13. Almestad E. Exploring explainable AI adoption in medical diagnosis and the empowering potential of collaboration. NTNU; 2023.
14. Moreno-Sanchez PA. Improvement of a prediction model for heart failure survival through explainable artificial intelligence. Front Cardiovasc Med. 2023;10:1219586.
15. Alam MN, Kaur M, Kabir MS. Explainable AI in healthcare: enhancing transparency and trust upon legal and ethical consideration. Int Res J Eng Technol. 2023;10(6):1–9.
16. Albahri AS, Duhaim AM, Fadhel MA, Alnoor A, Baqer NS, Alzubaidi L, et al. A systematic review of trustworthy and explainable artificial intelligence in healthcare: assessment of quality, bias risk, and data fusion. Inf Fusion. 2023;96:156.
17. De Laat PB. Algorithmic decision-making based on machine learning from big data: can transparency restore accountability? Philos Technol. 2018;31(4):525–41.
18. Baryannis G, Dani S, Antoniou G. Predicting supply chain risks using machine learning: the trade-off between performance and interpretability. Futur Gener Comput Syst. 2019;101:993–1004.
19. Dziugaite GK, Ben-David S, Roy DM. Enforcing interpretability and its statistical impacts: trade-offs between accuracy and interpretability. arXiv Prepr arXiv201013764. 2020.
20. Freitas AA. Automated machine learning for studying the trade-off between predictive accuracy and interpretability. In: International cross-domain conference for machine learning and knowledge extraction. Springer; 2019. p. 48–66.
21. Antoniadi AM, Du Y, Guendouz Y, Wei L, Mazo C, Becker BA, et al. Current challenges and future opportunities for XAI in machine learning-based clinical decision support systems: a systematic review. Appl Sci. 2021;11(11):5088.
22. Khanna S, Srivastava S. AI governance in healthcare: Explainability standards, safety protocols, and human-AI interactions dynamics in contemporary medical AI systems. Empir Quests Manag Essences. 2021;1(1):130–43.

23. Amoroso N, Pomarico D, Fanizzi A, Didonna V, Giotta F, La Forgia D, et al. A roadmap towards breast cancer therapies supported by explainable artificial intelligence. Appl Sci. 2021;11(11):4881.
24. Nagaraj P, Muneeswaran V, Dharanidharan A, Balananthanan K, Arunkumar M, Rajkumar C. A prediction and recommendation system for diabetes mellitus using XAI-based lime explainer. In: 2022 international conference on sustainable computing and data communication systems (ICSCDS). IEEE; 2022. p. 1472–8.
25. El-Sappagh S, Alonso JM, Islam SMR, Sultan AM, Kwak KS. A multilayer multimodal detection and prediction model based on explainable artificial intelligence for Alzheimer's disease. Sci Rep. 2021;11(1):2660.
26. Shad HA, Rahman QA, Asad NB, Bakshi AZ, Mursalin SMF, Reza MT, et al. Exploring Alzheimer's disease prediction with XAI in various neural network models. In: TENCON 2021–2021 IEEE region 10 conference (TENCON). IEEE; 2021. p. 720–5.
27. Kavya R, Christopher J, Panda S, Lazarus YB. Machine learning and XAI approaches for allergy diagnosis. Biomed Signal Process Control. 2021;69:102681.
28. Wu H, Chen W, Xu S, Xu B. Counterfactual supporting facts extraction for explainable medical record based diagnosis with graph network. In: Proceedings of the 2021 conference of the north American chapter of the association for computational linguistics: human language technologies; 2021. p. 1942–55.
29. Zhang Y, Weng Y, Lund J. Applications of explainable artificial intelligence in diagnosis and surgery. Diagnostics. 2022;12(2)
30. Coeckelbergh M. AI ethics. Mit Press; 2020.
31. Iserson KV. Informed consent for artificial intelligence in emergency medicine: a practical guide. Am J Emerg Med. 2024;76:225–30.
32. Srivastava G, Jhaveri RH, Bhattacharya S, Pandya S, Maddikunta PKR, Yenduri G, et al. XAI for cybersecurity: state of the art, challenges, open issues and future directions. arXiv Prepr arXiv220603585. 2022.
33. González-Sendino R, Serrano E, Bajo J, Novais P. A Review of Bias and Fairness in Artificial Intelligence. 2023.
34. González-Sendino R, Serrano E, Bajo J. Mitigating bias in artificial intelligence: fair data generation via causal models for transparent and explainable decision-making. Futur Gener Comput Syst. 2024;155:384.
35. Chuan CH, Sun R, Tian S, Tsai WHS. EXplainable artificial intelligence (XAI) for facilitating recognition of algorithmic bias: an experiment from imposed users' perspectives. Telematics Inform. 2024;91:102135.
36. Ferrara E. Fairness and bias in artificial intelligence: a brief survey of sources, impacts, and mitigation strategies. Science. 2023;6(1):3.
37. Kamishima T, Akaho S, Sakuma J. Fairness-aware learning through regularization approach. In: 2011 IEEE 11th international conference on data mining workshops. IEEE; 2011. p. 643–50.
38. Wang Z, Dong X, Xue H, Zhang Z, Chiu W, Wei T, et al. Fairness-aware adversarial perturbation towards bias mitigation for deployed deep models. In: Proceedings of the IEEE/CVF conference on computer vision and pattern recognition; 2022. p. 10379–88.
39. Aïvodji U, Bidet F, Gambs S, Ngueveu RC, Tapp A. Local data debiasing for fairness based on generative adversarial training. Algorithms. 2021;14(3):87.
40. Brunner T, Diehl F, Le MT, Knoll A. Guessing smart: biased sampling for efficient black-box adversarial attacks. In: Proceedings of the IEEE/CVF international conference on computer vision; 2019. p. 4958–66.
41. Shi L, Rahman R, Melamed E, Gwizdka J, Rousseau JF, Ding Y. Using explainable AI to cross-validate socio-economic disparities among Covid-19 patient mortality. AMIA Summits Transl Sci Proc. 2023;2023:477.
42. Jiang W, Pardos ZA. Towards equity and algorithmic fairness in student grade prediction. In: Proceedings of the 2021 AAAI/ACM conference on AI, ethics, and society; 2021. p. 608–17.

43. Lahoti P, Beutel A, Chen J, Lee K, Prost F, Thain N, et al. Fairness without demographics through adversarially reweighted learning. Adv Neural Inf Process Syst. 2020;33:728–40.
44. Denton E, Hutchinson B, Mitchell M, Gebru T, Zaldivar A. Image counterfactual sensitivity analysis for detecting unintended bias. arXiv Prepr arXiv190606439. 2019.
45. Di Stefano PG, Hickey JM, Vasileiou V. Counterfactual fairness: removing direct effects through regularization. arXiv Prepr arXiv200210774. 2020.
46. Gong S, Liu X, Jain AK. Mitigating face recognition bias via group adaptive classifier. In: Proceedings of the IEEE/CVF conference on computer vision and pattern recognition; 2021. p. 3414–24.
47. Baniecki H, Biecek P. Adversarial attacks and defenses in explainable artificial intelligence: a survey. Inf Fusion. 2024;107:102303.
48. Shneiderman B. Bridging the gap between ethics and practice: guidelines for reliable, safe, and trustworthy human-centered AI systems. ACM Trans Interact Intell Syst. 2020;10(4):1–31.
49. Irwin RS, Richardson ND. Patient-focused care: using the right tools. Chest. 2006;130(1):73S–82S.
50. Schoonderwoerd TAJ, Jorritsma W, Neerincx MA, Van Den Bosch K. Human-centered XAI: developing design patterns for explanations of clinical decision support systems. Int J Hum Comput Stud. 2021;154:102684.
51. Amann J, Blasimme A, Vayena E, Frey D, Madai VI, Consortium P. Explainability for artificial intelligence in healthcare: a multidisciplinary perspective. BMC Med Inform Decis Mak. 2020;20:1–9.
52. Manresa-Yee C, Roig-Maimó MF, Ramis S, Mas-Sansó R. Advances in XAI: explanation interfaces in healthcare. In: Handbook of artificial intelligence in healthcare: Vol 2: practicalities and prospects. Springer; 2021. p. 357–69.
53. Kim M, Kim S, Kim J, Song TJ, Kim Y. Do stakeholder needs differ?-designing stakeholder-tailored explainable artificial intelligence (XAI) interfaces. Int J Hum Comput Stud. 2024;181:103160.

Transparent Models in Healthcare: Enhancing Decision Support Through Explainability

Alfredo Cuzzocrea, Francesco Folino, Luigi Pontieri, Pietro Sabatino, and Maryam Samami

Contents

Abstract This chapter introduces a framework employing inherently explainable Machine Learning models to provide intuitive global explanations for medical diagnostics. Our proposal uses a transparent approach based on *Soft Decision Trees* (SDTs) that offers direct insights into its decision-making processes, eliminating the need for post hoc explanation methods. SDTs combine the hierarchical structure of decision trees with the representational power of neural networks, allowing them to capture complex data patterns while maintaining interpretability. In the context of healthcare analytics, we apply SDTs to a classification task. The model is trained end-to-end using mini-batch gradient descent to minimize a cross-entropy loss, encouraging balanced hierarchical data partitioning. An ANOVA-based feature selection technique is implemented to reduce model complexity and enhance

A. Cuzzocrea · M. Samami
iDEA Lab, University of Calabria, Rende, CS, Italy
e-mail: alfredo.cuzzocrea@unical.it; maryam.samami@unical.it

F. Folino (✉) · L. Pontieri · P. Sabatino
ICAR-CNR, Rende, CS, Italy
e-mail: francesco.folino@icar.cnr.it; luigi.pontieri@icar.cnr.it; pietro.sabatino@icar.cnr.it

R. Ortale et al. (eds.), *Explainable Machine Intelligence in Healthcare*,
https://doi.org/10.1007/978-3-031-91379-2_2

interpretability. We tested our methodology on a dataset from a healthcare scenario, demonstrating that SDTs effectively provide precise and understandable diagnostic predictions. The findings emphasize the role of explainable artificial intelligence in enhancing trust and cooperation in healthcare decision-making.

Keywords Machine learning · Soft decision trees · Explainable AI · Clinical DSSs · Healthcare analytics · Predictive modeling

1 Introduction

In healthcare, where multiple professionals such as nurses, clinicians, and administrative staff collaborate, decision-making is a critical and complex process [24]. These decisions, whether made individually or collectively, are intensive in knowledge and span various clinical activities, including triage, diagnosis, prognosis, and treatment, as well as in areas like surveillance and prehospital care [4, 14]. The diversity in the required skill levels and the urgency of these decisions highlight the need for adequate support systems.

Artificial Intelligence (AI), specifically through advances in Machine Learning (ML), has significantly impacted healthcare, providing robust solutions that have evolved since the 1970s [1, 23]. Recent developments in ML research, coupled with the proliferation of healthcare-specific information systems, data standards, and intelligent medical devices, have propelled the integration of AI techniques in healthcare, fueling expectations for a technological revolution in this sector [7].

ML tools can potentially extract meaningful predictive models from extensive historical data, aiding healthcare providers by highlighting critical insights that might not be immediately apparent. Numerous studies have demonstrated the efficacy of ML in deriving predictive models from electronic health record (EHR) data to support decisions in triage or diagnosis, aiming to minimize errors and promote personalized patient care [13]. Furthermore, ML can enhance resource allocation decisions and improve operational efficiency within healthcare settings by predicting demands for critical resources or the outcomes of medical procedures [3].

Despite these advantages, the application of ML in clinical settings faces significant hurdles, primarily due to the complexity and opacity of many ML models, which limits their acceptance and utility in practice [7, 12]. This backdrop sets the stage for this paper, which focuses on enhancing clinical decision-making through interpretable ML models.

The current healthcare landscape still favors traditional decision support methods that healthcare professionals are familiar with, such as risk estimation models developed by domain experts and validated through long-standing usage in clinical practice [5]. These models, including indices like the LACE index for assessing readmission risks, are generally simple, focusing on key risk factors and facilitating ease of understanding and integration with clinical workflows [19, 27]. However, their limited capacity for personalized predictions and difficulty integrating with

EHR systems have highlighted the need for more adaptable and transparent solutions [26].

Conversely, while ML models offer more nuanced insights into patient data, thereby supporting personalized medicine, their "black-box" nature often precludes their acceptance by healthcare professionals who demand transparency and adherence to ethical standards [16]. This necessitates a shift toward inherently interpretable models, like Soft Decision Trees (SDTs), which balance the need for accuracy with interpretability in clinical decision support [9].

Our approach, therefore, leverages SDTs to construct interpretable prediction models that are precise and intuitive to healthcare providers. Unlike traditional decision trees (DTs), SDTs facilitate an end-to-end training process. In addition, the approach integrates (i) different kinds of attribution-like explanations, specifically conceived to help the user evaluate the actual and potential impact of each data feature on a model prediction and (ii) a feature selection mechanism, which can be exploited in a preprocessing phase to obtain simpler classification models and explanations, which are both easier to interpret and more suitable for rapid, energy-efficient computations essential in fast-paced medical settings.

Contribution
This chapter's contributions are twofold. First, we present a comprehensive framework that employs inherently explainable ML models, focusing on implementing SDTs that provide global, intuitive explanations suitable for medical diagnostics. Second, we pragmatically examine this approach using real-life healthcare data, illustrating its potential to impact diagnostic outcomes significantly. The findings emphasize explainable AI's role in enhancing healthcare decision-making and strengthening the collaboration between AI systems and medical professionals.

2 Related Work

The development of Clinical Decision Support Systems (CDSS) to assist healthcare professionals has a well-established history. Initial work on systems to aid clinical decision-making, particularly in diagnosis and treatment, began over 50 years ago [5]. In recent years, ML advances have driven further progress in enhancing clinical decision processes, providing more powerful analytical tools.

Traditional models for clinical risk assessment, such as the LACE index [27] for predicting readmission and early mortality, and domain-specific Logistic Regression (LR) models, have played a significant role in risk evaluation for many years [19]. These models typically utilize multivariate regression techniques to analyze clinical factors, assigning risk scores based on regression coefficients [22]. Despite their long-standing use, these models face limitations due to their reliance on linear relationships between predictors and outcomes, which can reduce their effectiveness in providing personalized predictions [2, 16].

More sophisticated ML-based approaches have emerged for risk and outcome prediction in response to these limitations. Techniques that leverage deep neural networks, random forests, and gradient-boosted trees often outperform traditional score-based models by capturing complex, nonlinear relationships within the data [13, 25]. However, the increased complexity of these models has raised concerns around interpretability, making it challenging for clinicians to fully trust or understand the predictions generated by these systems [6, 28].

To improve transparency, research has focused on post hoc explanation methods that attempt to clarify the predictions of these "black-box" models [11]. However, debate continues regarding the reliability of these explanations in accurately representing the internal mechanisms of the underlying models [20, 29]. As a result, attention has shifted toward inherently interpretable models, such as decision trees, which balance interpretability with performance. These simpler models, however, often lack the predictive power of more advanced methods [7].

Among these approaches, SDTs have gained traction due to their ability to offer both interpretability and flexibility. Unlike traditional decision trees, which make hard decisions at each node, SDTs use probabilistic soft splits, allowing the model to combine information from multiple branches. This results in smoother decision boundaries and can lead to better generalization compared to standard decision trees [15]. SDTs have been applied in various domains, including healthcare, where they provide a compromise between accuracy and interpretability, which is critical in clinical decision-making [10].

By offering a more flexible framework, SDTs can handle uncertainty and variability in patient data more effectively than rigid decision trees. This has proven helpful in complex scenarios, such as predicting patient outcomes based on multiple, potentially conflicting factors. Studies have shown that SDTs can outperform both traditional decision trees and simple logistic regression models in terms of predictive accuracy while still offering the transparency required for clinical use [10, 15]. Additionally, their interpretability makes them well suited for integration into CDSS, where clinicians need understandable and reliable models.

For example, SDTs have been applied to clinical scenarios such as predicting patient survival rates in critical care settings. The smooth transitions between decision paths in these models help account for nuances in patient data often overlooked by conventional decision trees. Furthermore, SDTs can be enhanced through techniques such as feature selection, helping to mitigate information loss and improve model performance [17, 21]. This makes them a promising approach for balancing the trade-off between interpretability and accuracy in clinical decision support.

3 Problem and Solution Framework: Soft Decision Tree Classifier for Binary Classification

This section defines the binary classification problem addressed in this work and the model adopted to tackle it.

3.1 *Problem Description*

The problem at hand is a supervised binary classification task. We are given a dataset where each instance consists of a feature vector representing the characteristics of an observation, along with a binary label indicating its class. The objective is to develop a model that can accurately classify unseen examples based on these features.

In healthcare scenarios, classification tasks often involve predicting patient outcomes, diagnoses, or risk levels based on patient data, such as demographics, medical history, and clinical measurements. These predictions must be reliable, but equally important, they must be explainable. In this context, the model must be accurate and interpretable by clinicians, who must be able to trust the model's decisions and understand the reasoning behind them.

Overfitting is a significant concern in such tasks. A too complex model may perform well on training data but fail to generalize to new, unseen cases. This is particularly problematic in healthcare, where overfitting could lead to incorrect or overly confident predictions about new patients, potentially leading to harmful decisions. To address this, feature selection is applied to remove irrelevant or redundant information, simplifying the model and improving its generalization ability.

To tackle this binary classification problem, we adopt a SDT model. SDTs balance the interpretability of traditional decision trees and the flexibility of more complex models like neural networks. This makes them particularly suitable for healthcare, where accuracy and explainability are paramount.

3.2 *Soft Decision Tree Classifier*

In healthcare, the need for inherently interpretable models cannot be overstated. Clinicians must be able to trust the predictions made by a model, especially when these predictions may inform critical decisions. Models that operate as "black boxes"—producing accurate but opaque predictions—can undermine trust and hinder their practical adoption in clinical settings.

Traditional decision trees are popular due to their simplicity and transparency, as they provide clear, step-by-step rules for classification. However, these models often struggle with complex data patterns, leading to reduced accuracy. On the other hand,

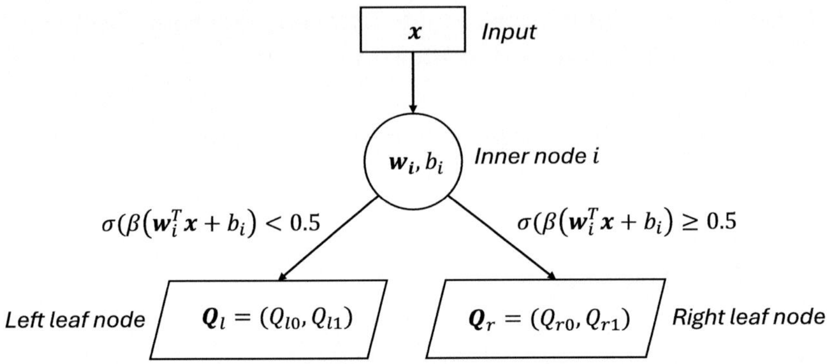

Fig. 1 An example SDT featuring a single inner node and two leaf nodes

models like deep neural networks, while more powerful, lack the interpretability needed in sensitive applications like healthcare.

Soft Decision Trees strike a balance between these two extremes. They maintain a tree-like structure, which is familiar and interpretable, but introduce soft, probabilistic splits instead of hard, deterministic ones. This makes them flexible enough to model complex, nonlinear relationships in the data while preserving a level of transparency crucial for clinical use. With SDTs, each decision is not a rigid "yes" or "no" but a probability that an observation belongs to a particular branch, allowing for more nuanced decision-making. A representation of a simplified SDT featuring a single inner node and two leaf nodes is shown in Fig. 1.

Each SDT consists of *inner nodes* and *leaf nodes*. Inner nodes are responsible for the decision-making process, where a probabilistic split is made based on the input feature vector $\mathbf{x}$. This decision is controlled by the learned weight vector $\mathbf{w}_i$, bias b_i, and an essential parameter, β. The soft decision at each inner node i is represented by the sigmoid function $\sigma(\beta(\mathbf{w}_i^T\mathbf{x} + b_i))$. The role of β is crucial as it adjusts the "sharpness" of the decision boundary; higher values of β lead to more deterministic (hard) decisions, whereas lower values make the splits softer and more probabilistic. This flexibility in decision-making is essential in healthcare, where patient data often contains uncertainty or overlaps between conditions.

The outputs of the inner nodes direct the input toward either the left or right leaf nodes, representing the final predictions. Each leaf node contains a probability distribution over the possible outcome classes, denoted by $Q_\ell = (Q_{\ell 0}, Q_{\ell 1})$ for the left leaf and $Q_r = (Q_{r0}, Q_{r1})$ for the right leaf in the example in Fig. 1. The tree computes a final probability distribution based on the path from the root to the leaf.

3.2.1 Differences from Classical Decision Trees

In a traditional decision tree, each internal node applies a hard split based on a feature value. Based on a fixed threshold, this deterministic split sends an instance to the left or the right branch. While easy to interpret, this rigidity often leads to poor generalization of new data, particularly in healthcare scenarios where data can be noisy or complex. Hard splits can cause overfitting, especially when the model is deep, making overly confident decisions based on slight variations in the data.

Soft Decision Trees, by contrast, make probabilistic decisions at each internal node. Rather than routing an instance strictly down one path, an SDT assigns probabilities to all possible branches. This allows each instance to be distributed across multiple branches, reflecting the inherent uncertainty in medical data. For example, a patient might exhibit symptoms that place them near the boundary between two diagnoses; an SDT can account for this uncertainty by partially classifying them into both categories, reflecting the true complexity of the decision.

This probabilistic approach reduces overfitting by avoiding rigid decisions and improves generalization by allowing the model to learn smoother decision boundaries. This flexibility can lead to more reliable predictions when dealing with heterogeneous patient data in a healthcare setting.

3.2.2 Training of Soft Decision Trees

SDTs are trained using gradient-based optimization methods, such as mini-batch gradient descent, in contrast to traditional decision trees' greedy, stepwise approach. This joint optimization process ensures that all tree parts are optimized simultaneously, improving the model's overall performance and cohesion. The objective is to minimize the cross-entropy loss, which measures how well the predicted probabilities match the actual class labels.

This training process is beneficial in healthcare, where data is often limited or imbalanced. The global optimization of the tree's parameters ensures that the model can still learn robust patterns without overfitting, even with small or unbalanced datasets. By optimizing all nodes together, SDTs avoid the local optima that traditional trees might fall into when splitting the data at each node in isolation.

3.2.3 Regularization in Soft Decision Trees

A core feature of SDTs is their use of regularization to prevent overfitting, which is critical in healthcare, where the consequences of incorrect predictions can be severe. SDTs include a regularization term that penalizes unbalanced data splits, ensuring that the tree does not become overly specialized in certain branches. This regularization encourages more balanced data partitions, leading to a more robust model that generalizes better to new patients. By penalizing unbalanced splits, the model avoids over-relying on a few strong features, which is often a problem in healthcare datasets where specific clinical measurements might dominate the decision-making process. Regularization ensures that the model considers a broader range of features, leading to more reliable and interpretable decisions.

3.2.4 Interpretability of Soft Decision Trees

SDTs are particularly suitable for healthcare because of their inherent interpretability. Every decision in an SDT can be traced back to a combination of feature weights and probabilities, providing a clear rationale for the final classification. In healthcare, where transparency is critical, this interpretability allows clinicians to understand the prediction, confidence, and reasoning behind it.

Furthermore, SDTs use probabilistic splits, so naturally dealing with prediction uncertainty. In many healthcare applications, decisions are not binary: Patients may exhibit symptoms that place them near the boundary between two possible diagnoses. By providing a clinician with a probability distribution over the classes, SDTs give her more nuanced information to base her decision on.

3.3 Feature Selection

In general, feature selection is a powerful means for curbing the complexity and machine learning models while possibly reducing the risk of overfitting, especially in high-dimensional spaces.

In this work, we resort to ANOVA (Analysis of Variance), a popular classic method for identifying features significantly affecting a target variable. In this method, for each feature j, the F-statistic is calculated as follows:

$$F_j = \frac{\text{Between-group variability}}{\text{Within-group variability}} = \frac{\sum_{k=1}^{K} n_k(\bar{x}_{kj} - \bar{x}_j)^2/(K-1)}{\sum_{k=1}^{K}\sum_{i \in \text{group } k}(x_{ij} - \bar{x}_{kj})^2/(n-K)} \tag{1}$$

where n_k is the number of samples in class k, $\bar{x}_{kj}$ is the mean of feature j for class k, $\bar{x}_j$ is the overall mean of feature j, and n is the total number of observations. Eventually, features with high F-values are considered more discriminative and retained when constructing a model for the data.

4 Experiments

This section evaluates the effectiveness and explainability of various machine learning models using three widely available clinical datasets, highlighting their relevance in healthcare analytics. This comparison between interpretable models and their more complex, opaque alternatives demonstrates their practical value in medical environments. The assessment explores the advantages and limitations of each model type, offering an in-depth appraisal of their predictive power concerning clinical outcomes.

4.1 Experimental Setup

4.1.1 Case Study

The `Heart` disease dataset available on the Kaggle[1] repository, initially introduced in [8], has been an important resource in numerous studies for the development of predictive models and the examination of risk factors linked to heart disease. Originating from four databases—Cleveland, Hungary, Switzerland, and Long Beach V—this dataset incorporates data from 1,025 patients and features 76 attributes. However, most research has focused on a core subset of 13 critical attributes. These attributes, encompassing demographic information, blood test results, and outcomes of stress tests, are vital for assessing the risk of heart disease in individuals.

In more detail, the 13 critical attributes within this dataset are the following: "age" (age in years), "sex" (where 1 denotes male and 0 female), "cp" (chest pain type, indicating the severity/type of chest pain), "trestbps" (resting blood pressure in mm Hg upon hospital admission), "chol" (serum cholesterol in mg/dl), "fbs" (fasting blood sugar, with values greater than 120 mg/dl marked as 1 for true, and 0 for false), "restecg" (resting electrocardiographic results), "thalach" (maximum heart rate achieved), "exang" (exercise-induced angina, with 1 for yes and 0 for no), "oldpeak" (ST depression induced by exercise relative to rest), "slope" (slope of the peak exercise ST segment), "ca" (number of major vessels identified by fluoroscopy, ranging from 0 to 3), and "thal" (status of thalassemia categorized as normal, fixed defect, or reversible defect).

In terms of data preparation, essential steps undertaken include the addressing of missing values, along with the normalization or standardization of numerical attributes and the encoding of categorical features. These procedures ensure the dataset is optimally configured for analysis via machine learning models.

The dataset's target variable "target," meant to indicate the presence of heart disease, was initially set to 0 (no disease) and values ranging from 1 to 4 representing varying degrees of severity. However, for the sake of simplification and to support comparative analysis, numerous studies—including ours—have opted to recode this variable into a binary outcome: 0 for the absence of disease and 1 for its presence. This recoding strategy results in a balanced dataset, with the presence of heart disease (label 1) representing approximately 51.3% of all possible cases.

4.1.2 Competitors and Baseline Models

This analysis compares the soft decision tree approach with two other models: a Multi-layer Perceptron (MLP) and an LR. The MLP, known for its capability to model (nonlinear) complex patterns through multiple hidden layers, serves as an upper-bound reference model. This comparison is instrumental in assessing the

[1] https://www.kaggle.com/datasets/johnsmith88/heart-disease-dataset

effectiveness of our approach against a high-performing, albeit non-explainable, black-box model.

On the other hand, the interpretable LR model, chosen as a baseline, exhibits a simpler architecture. Each input feature connects to each output class through a weight, plus a bias for each class. The model's simplicity and the compactness of its explanations make LR highly suitable for applications like clinical "risk calculators," underscoring its reliability and relevance as a comparative baseline in our study.

Comparing SDT to these models entails considering distinct aspects. While the comparison with MLP should help gauge the maximal performance one might achieve (albeit without any explanation), the comparison with LR should show a more favorable trade-off for SDT between effectiveness and explainability.

4.1.3 Test Procedure and Parameter Settings

This study employs *Python 3.11.7* and *PyTorch 2.1.2* to implement the three distinct approaches in our analysis: SDT, MLP, and LR. In particular, the SDT code is adapted from an existing public repository on GitHub.[2]

The architecture of the SDT was configured with varying numbers of inner nodes, specifically $D \in \{4, 6\}$, to explore the impact of model size on performance, while the parameter β, in our implementation, was dynamically learned during training to optimize decision boundaries.

In contrast, MLP is structured with two hidden layers containing 32 and 16 neurons, respectively, and uses a RELU activation function. The LR model is simplified to a single linear layer. All models employ a softmax function to output the probabilities of binary class assignments (0 or 1) at their respective decision boundaries.

All models were trained and tested for experimental consistency across identical dataset configurations and hyperparameter settings. Each dataset was randomly divided into training and test sets, with the test set comprising 20% of the total data. A further 20% of the training data was segregated to form a validation set used for model selection based on the lowest validation loss. To mitigate statistical biases, this process was replicated across ten distinct runs using ten unique random seeds, with results averaged to ensure robustness.

Common training parameters were standardized across all models. We set the training to a maximum of 40 epochs, a batch size of 32, and a learning rate of 0.01, using the Adam optimizer for all approaches.

Finally, an ANOVA-based feature selection technique was implemented to reduce the input features, enhancing both model efficacy and interpretability (see Sect. 3.3). This reduction halved the original number of features from d to $\lfloor \frac{d}{2} \rfloor$, focusing on the features most relevant to the target class label.

2 https://github.com/kimhc6028/soft-decision-tree/

4.1.4 Evaluation Metrics

In healthcare predictive analytics, binary classification tasks are instrumental for distinguishing between two primary outcomes: a “standard” class, representing expected or normal outcomes (e.g., healthy individuals or standard discharge scenarios like “Release A”), and a “non-standard” class, indicating the presence of a condition requiring attention (e.g., disease presence or discharge scenarios other than “Release A”). This differentiation is crucial for accurately identifying cases requiring further medical evaluation or specific interventions.

The effectiveness of predictive models in this context is evaluated through various metrics, each shedding light on different facets of the model’s diagnostic or predictive accuracy. These evaluations hinge on four key outcomes: *True Positives (TP)*, nonstandard cases correctly identified, *True Negatives (TN)*, standard cases accurately recognized, *False Positives (FP)*, standard cases mistakenly flagged as nonstandard, and *False Negatives (FN)*, nonstandard cases incorrectly classified as standard. Striking the right balance between correctly identifying nonstandard cases and minimizing incorrect classifications is essential for optimizing patient care and resource management.

Significative metrics utilized in healthcare analytics include:

- *Accuracy* (ACC) quantifies the model’s overall correctness, expressed as $(TP + TN)/(TP + TN + FP + FN)$. By returning the fraction of correct predictions, this metric provides a measure of the model’s reliability. However, accuracy must be used cautiously in the case of imbalanced classes.
- *Area Under the ROC Curve* (AUC) assesses the model’s discriminative ability between standard and nonstandard classes across varying thresholds. A higher AUC reflects better performance in distinguishing between the two outcomes, crucial for ensuring accurate identification without excessive FP.
- *Precision* (PREC), computed as $TP/(TP + FP)$, emphasizes the model’s accuracy in predicting nonstandard outcomes, aiming to reduce the misclassification of standard cases as nonstandard.
- *Sensitivity* (SENS), also known as *Recall*, calculated as $TP/(TP + FN)$, measures the model’s ability to detect all actual nonstandard cases, critical for not missing any cases requiring intervention.
- *F1-score* (F1) integrates Precision (the accuracy of identifying nonstandard cases) and Sensitivity (the model’s completeness in capturing all nonstandard cases) into a single metric, calculated as $2 \cdot (\texttt{PREC} \cdot \texttt{SENS})/(\texttt{PREC} + \texttt{SENS})$. This metric is especially relevant when the consequences of misclassifications are significant, ensuring a balance between Sensitivity and Precision.

Collectively, these metrics offer comprehensive insights into a model’s performance in healthcare settings, highlighting the importance of a multifaceted evaluation approach. However, in our clinical setting, where early detection of diabetes, cardiovascular diseases, and breast cancer is critical, SENS can be considered the reference metric because it ensures the model effectively identifies all potential cases, minimizing the risk of overlooking patients who require urgent medical attention.

4.2 Test Results

In the context of healthcare-related datasets, our study focuses on a comparative analysis of SDT, MLP, and LR models, with a particular emphasis on performance and explainability—both critical for medical applications where predictions must be interpretable by healthcare practitioners. As shown in Table 1, the results are based on experiments conducted on the `Heart` dataset.

From the examination of performance metrics in Table 1, SDTs configured with six inner nodes ($D = 6$) and without feature selection outperform LR in `SENS`, a key metric in our medical setting, with a notable 6.4% margin. SDT also outperforms the nonlinear, non-explainable MLP in `SENS`, with a 3.0% improvement. These results highlight SDT's superiority in sensitivity, which is particularly important in healthcare scenarios where minimizing false negatives is critical.

While MLP performs similarly regarding overall accuracy, it lacks the explainability inherent in SDTs. MLPs, despite their predictive power, require post hoc methods such as LIME [18] to provide explanations, whereas SDTs offer transparent decision paths that naturally reflect the decision-making process. This interpretability is essential in medical contexts, where understanding the rationale behind a diagnosis is as important as the accuracy of the prediction itself.

Although SDTs are more complex than LR, this is counterbalanced by their improved predictive performance. In medical applications where reliable and interpretable outcomes are essential, SDTs stand out as a strong option, providing both accurate and explainable predictions.

When analyzing SDTs with a reduced depth, specifically $D = 4$, a decline in performance is observed compared to the $D = 6$ configuration, as expected. On

Table 1 Performance results obtained by the proposed SDT model, the black-box MLP, and a baseline model LR on the real-life `Heart`. These results are meant to help investigate the effects of varying the depth of SDTs (denoted by D) and input data dimension (denoted by d), considering scenarios both with and without feature selection. Best results are shown in bold

Model	d	D	Explainability	ACC	AUC	F1	PREC	SENS
SDT	13	6	YES	**0.873**	**0.938**	**0.873**	**0.844**	**0.912**
SDT		4	YES	0.846	0.917	0.845	0.830	0.864
MLP		–	NO	0.859	**0.938**	0.859	0.835	0.886
LR		–	YES	0.810	0.895	0.814	0.775	0.857
SDT	6	6	YES	0.818	0.890	0.816	0.762	0.910
SDT		4	YES	0.808	0.879	0.807	0.754	0.903
MLP		–	NO	0.829	0.897	0.836	0.788	0.892
LR		–	YES	0.786	0.867	0.794	0.748	0.848

average, there is a slight drop in performance metrics, including a 1.4% decrease in SENS. However, even in this simplified form, SDTs still outperform LR by a consistent margin, demonstrating their ability to capture complex patterns in the data more effectively than linear models. Furthermore, the performance gap between SDT ($D = 4$) and MLP remains narrow, with SDT lagging by only 1%, underscoring its competitive predictive capability even with reduced complexity.

Regarding the impact of feature selection, halving the number of input features ($d = 6$) affects SDT performance to some extent on the Heart dataset, where the reduction in the feature set leads to a noticeable decline in overall performance. This suggests that while SDTs can handle smaller feature spaces, the Heart dataset may be more sensitive to feature reduction, potentially requiring more features to capture the nuances in patient data. Nonetheless, SDTs maintain a strong balance between accuracy and interpretability, even operating on a streamlined feature set.

In summary, SDTs combine the good performance of nonlinear models with the simplicity and explainability of linear ones. The best results are achieved with $D = 6$ inner nodes and the complete feature set, but even with $D = 4$ SDTs stay competitive. This makes SDTs particularly well suited for clinical applications where both interpretability and high predictive performance are essential.

4.3 Analyzing Explanations of SDT Predictions

To evaluate the interpretability and reliability of SDT predictions, we focus on a specific model, denoted as M^{ex}, generated by setting the tree depth to $D = 6$ and using the entire feature set ($d = 13$) of the Heart dataset. This model exhibits superior predictive performance compared to its competitors, as shown in Table 1.

As to the interpretability of the predictions obtained and the interestingness of the associated explanations, let us consider the case of a (randomly selected) test instance $\mathbf{x}^{ex}$, the normalized features of which are shown in Table 2. This instance, belonging to class "1," was rightly assigned to this class by M^{ex}.

Table 3 shows all the parameters of the model associated with the internal nodes along the decision path taken by $\mathbf{x}^{ex}$, while the classification of $\mathbf{x}^{ex}$ by M^{ex}, involving traversing six internal nodes, is illustrated in Table 4. At each of these nodes, the decision to move left or right was taken by summing up the weighted feature-wise values $v_0, \ldots, v_{12}$ and the node's bias and multiplying the resulting *logit* value by a scaling factor (β); the probability of turning right was then computed by making the resulting value through a logistic function. Based on this probability, the direction of traversal was eventually chosen. In this computation, the trainable parameter β influences the sharpness of the decision boundary, and it can even reverse (when $beta < 0$) the direction indicated by the logit's sign.

From Table 4, it is clear that the values v_7 and v_{10} (i.e., the coefficient-multiplied features thalach and slope, respectively) play a crucial role in the routing decisions taken for $\mathbf{x}^{ex}$ within the SDT. Specifically, v_7 and v_{10} neatly affected four and three, respectively, of the routing decisions. In particular, v_7 is the term

Table 2 Features and corresponding normalized values for a test instance $\mathbf{x}^{ex}$ randomly selected from the `Heart` dataset

Feature	Name	Value	Description
0	age	0.687	Normalized age of the patient
1	sex	0.000	Gender of the patient (0 = female, 1 = male)
2	cp	0.000	Type of chest pain
3	trestbps	0.283	Resting blood pressure
4	chol	0.189	Serum cholesterol in mg/dl
5	fbs	0.000	Fasting blood sugar > 120 mg/dl (1 = true; 0 = false)
6	restecg	0.500	Resting electrocardiographic results
7	thalach	0.702	Maximum heart rate achieved
8	exang	0.000	Exercise-induced angina (1 = yes; 0 = no)
9	oldpeak	0.000	ST depression induced by exercise relative to rest
10	slope	1.000	The slope of the peak exercise ST segment
11	ca	0.000	Number of major vessels (0–3) colored by fluoroscopy
12	thal	0.667	Thalassemia ()

that contributed the most to the logit value at certain nodes. However, in some inner nodes, the direction suggested by v_7 was reversed due to the presence of a negative β value—this is, e.g., the case of node 1, where a "go-left" decision was eventually taken.

Conducting a finer-grain analysis, we note that values v_0 and v_6 (corresponding to features `age` and `restecg`) contributed appreciably at some decisions, particularly at nodes 4 and 5. Here, their opposing signs lead to more complex interactions, also influenced by the sign and magnitude of β. This intricate interplay between the feature-related terms and β highlights the flexibility of SDTs in capturing nuanced dependencies between the class variable and the data features.

5 Conclusion and Future Work

We have introduced a framework using SDTs to improve decision support in healthcare by enhancing explainability. SDTs merge the hierarchical structure of decision trees with the representational power of neural nets, allowing them to capture complex data patterns while enjoying the interpretability of decision trees. Through probabilistic splits and global optimization, SDTs offer more robust models that overcome limitations like overfitting and lacking global context.

Experiments demonstrated SDTs' ability to provide intuitive and transparent predictions, addressing the "black-box" nature of deep learning and promoting their trustworthy use in clinical settings. A comparative analysis with traditional models like logistic regressors and multilayer perceptrons showed SDTs' beneficial balance between performance and explainability.

Table 3 SDT model, M^{ex}, trained on the Heart dataset with all $d = 13$ features. For each inner node k along the decision path, the table presents the coefficients $(c_0, \ldots, c_{12})$ corresponding to each feature, along with the bias term and the inverse temperature parameter (β) for the logistic regressor learned at that node

k	c_0	c_1	c_2	c_3	c_4	c_5	c_6	c_7	c_8	c_9	c_{10}	c_{11}	c_{12}	Bias	β
1	0.16	−1.77	0.40	−0.71	−0.44	0.65	0.77	1.81	−0.54	−1.45	0.77	−3.72	−0.96	0.95	−4.86
2	−0.40	−0.84	−2.44	0.04	0.09	1.07	−0.73	0.96	2.82	−2.15	0.35	0.24	0.43	0.28	2.34
3	0.49	1.10	−0.99	0.78	0.54	−0.41	−0.56	−0.83	1.13	0.87	−0.80	1.86	0.50	−0.17	4.91
4	−1.23	−0.90	1.65	−0.85	−1.76	0.81	1.64	0.87	−0.51	0.63	0.37	−2.09	−0.46	0.24	−4.29
5	−0.55	−0.87	0.60	−0.24	−0.45	0.28	0.68	0.08	−0.09	−0.38	0.27	−0.42	−0.41	0.19	−2.06
6	0.18	0.17	0.55	0.27	0.12	0.10	0.50	0.61	−0.01	0.32	0.50	0.07	0.44	0.38	4.07

Table 4 Explanation of the decision path for the test instance $\mathbf{x}^{ex}$ using an SDT. For each inner node k, the table shows the multiplication of each feature value with the corresponding coefficient of M^{ex} (i.e., $v_i = c_i \cdot x_i^{ex}$, for $i = 0, \ldots, 12$), the bias, the β value, the probability computed at that node, and the decision (right or left child). The feature values with higher absolute magnitudes are shown in bold

k	v_0	v_1	v_2	v_3	v_4	v_5	v_6	v_7	v_8	v_9	v_{10}	v_{11}	v_{12}	Bias	β	Prob.	Decision
1	0.11	0.00	0.00	−0.20	−0.08	0.00	0.39	**1.27**	0.00	0.00	0.77	0.00	−0.64	**0.95**	−4.86	0.00	Left
2	−0.27	0.00	0.00	0.01	0.02	0.00	−0.37	**0.67**	0.00	0.00	**0.35**	0.00	0.29	0.28	2.34	0.91	Right
3	0.34	0.00	0.00	0.22	0.10	0.00	−0.28	**−0.58**	0.00	0.00	**−0.80**	0.00	0.33	−0.17	4.91	0.02	Left
4	**−0.85**	0.00	0.00	−0.24	−0.33	0.00	**0.82**	0.61	0.00	0.00	0.37	0.00	−0.31	0.24	−4.29	0.21	Left
5	**−0.38**	0.00	0.00	−0.07	−0.09	0.00	**0.34**	0.06	0.00	0.00	0.27	0.00	−0.27	0.19	−2.06	0.47	Left
6	0.12	0.00	0.00	0.08	0.02	0.00	0.25	**0.43**	0.00	0.00	**0.50**	0.00	0.29	0.38	4.07	1.00	Right

Future research includes exploiting pretrained neural net and integrating domain knowledge to guide the training of STD models and improve their interpretability and reliability. Specifically, accounting for clinical guidelines and domain expertise can better align the discovered models with medical practices, fostering more effective and trustworthy CDSs.

Acknowledgments This work was partly supported by *(i)* research project FAIR—Future AI Research—Spoke 9 (Directorial Decree No. 1243, August 2, 2022; PE 0000013; CUP B53C22003630006), under the NRRP (National Recovery and Resilience Plan) MUR program (Mission 4, Component 2 Investment 1.3) funded by the European Union—NextGenerationEU, and *(ii)* research project PINPOINT (exPlaInable kNowledge-aware PrOcess INTelligence), under program PRIN funded by Italian Ministry MUR (B27G22000160001).

References

1. Ali O, et al. A systematic literature review of artificial intelligence in the healthcare sector: Benefits, challenges, methodologies, and functionalities. J Innov Knowl. 2023;8(1):100333.
2. Allen LA, et al. Use of risk models to predict death in the next year among individual ambulatory patients with heart failure. JAMA Cardiol. 2017;2(4):435–41.
3. Alzu'bi A, Najadat H, Doulat W, Al-Shari O, Zhou L. Predicting the recurrence of breast cancer using machine learning algorithms. Multimed Tools Appl. 2021;80:13787–800.
4. Bashiri A, et al. Promotion of prehospital emergency care through clinical decision support systems: Opportunities and challenges. Clin Exp Emerg Med. 2019;6(4):288.
5. Belard A, et al. Precision diagnosis: A view of the clinical decision support systems (CDSS) landscape through the lens of critical care. J Clin Monit Comput. 2017;31:261–71.
6. Bharati S, Mondal MRH, Podder P. A review on explainable artificial intelligence for healthcare: Why, how, and when? IEEE Trans Artif Intell. 2023;5(4):1429–42.
7. Buchard A, Richens JG. Artificial intelligence for medical decisions. Cham: Springer; 2022. pp. 159–79.
8. Detrano R, et al. International application of a new probability algorithm for the diagnosis of coronary artery disease. Am J Cardiol. 1989;64(5):304–10.
9. Frosst N, Hinton G. Distilling a neural network into a soft decision tree. arXiv preprint arXiv:1711.09784. 2017.
10. Frosst N, Hinton G. Distilling a neural network into a soft decision tree. In: Proceedings of the 20th international conference on machine learning (ICML), Sydney. 2017. pp. 3–10.
11. Guidotti R, et al. A survey of methods for explaining black box models. ACM Comput Surv. 2018;51(5):1–42.
12. He X, Zheng X, Ding H. Existing barriers faced by and future design recommendations for direct-to-consumer health care artificial intelligence apps: Scoping review. J Med Internet Res. 2023;25:e50342.
13. Hobensack M, Song J, Scharp D, Bowles KH, Topaz M. Machine learning applied to electronic health record data in home healthcare: A scoping review. Int J Med Inform. 2023;170:104978.
14. Horn W. Ai in medicine on its way from knowledge-intensive to data-intensive systems. Artif Intell Med. 2001;23(1):5–12.
15. Irsoy O, Yildiz OT. Soft decision trees. In: Proceedings of the 21st international conference on pattern recognition (ICPR). 2012. pp. 1819–22.
16. Li Y, et al. Do population-level risk prediction models that use routinely collected health data reliably predict individual risks? Sci Rep. 2019;9(1):11222.

17. Ning Y, et al. A novel interpretable machine learning system to generate clinical risk scores: An application for predicting early mortality or unplanned readmission in a retrospective cohort study. PLOS Digit Health. 2022;1(6):1–20.
18. Ribeiro MT, Singh S, Guestrin C. Why should i trust you? Explaining the predictions of any classifier. In: Proceedings of the 22nd ACM SIGKDD international conference on knowledge discovery and data mining, San Francisco; 2016. pp. 1135–44.
19. Robinson R, Hudali T. The hospital score and lace index as predictors of 30 day readmission in a retrospective study at a university-affiliated community hospital. PeerJ. 2017;5:e3137
20. Slack D, Hilgard A, Singh S, Lakkaraju H. Reliable post hoc explanations: Modeling uncertainty in explainability. Adv Neural Inf Proces Syst. 2021;34:9391–404.
21. Su W, Bogdan M, Candes E. False discoveries occur early on the lasso path. Ann Stat. 2017;45(5):2133–50.
22. Sullivan LM, Massaro JM, Sr D'Agostino RB. Presentation of multivariate data for clinical use: The Framingham study risk score functions. Stat Med. 2004;23(10):1631–60.
23. Sutton RT, et al. An overview of clinical decision support systems: Benefits, risks, and strategies for success. NPJ Digit Med. 2020;3(1):17.
24. Tien JM, Goldschmidt-Clermont PJ. Healthcare: A complex service system. J. Syst Sci Syst Eng. 2009;18:257–82.
25. Twick I, Zahavi G, Benvenisti H, Rubinstein R, Woods MS, Berkenstadt H, Nissan A, Hosgor E, Assaf D. Towards interpretable, medically grounded, EMR-based risk prediction models. Sci Rep. 2022;12(1):9990.
26. Van Hee K, Schonenberg H, Serebrenik A, Sidorova N, Van Der Werf JM. Adaptive workflows for healthcare information systems. In: Business process management workshops, revised selected papers, Milano; 2008. pp. 359–70.
27. Van Walraven C, et al. Derivation and validation of an index to predict early death or unplanned readmission after discharge from hospital to the community. CMAJ. 2010;182(6):551–7.
28. Watson DS, et al. Clinical applications of machine learning algorithms: Beyond the black box. BMJ. 2019;364:l886.
29. Zhou Y, Booth S, Ribeiro MT, Shah J. Do feature attribution methods correctly attribute features? In: Proceedings of AAAI conference on artificial intelligence (AAAI'22), Virtual event; 2022. pp. 9623–33.

Improving Explanation Measures Inside the Decision-Making Process to Increase the Potential of AI Applications in Healthcare

Luka Poslon and Anto Čartolovni

Contents

Abstract The application of AI in healthcare sets a greater emphasis on pattern recognition for triaging, screening, classification, reporting cases, and other tasks than in other human endeavors. As a result, the outcome of AI predictions in healthcare frequently requires human approval or decision-making. Given that different users have varying backgrounds and levels of knowledge, it may not always be necessary to fully explain the underlying principles of AI application technologies in the healthcare sector to all users. However, when applying moral and legal guidelines to AI systems that comply with explainability and transparency standards, trustworthy data foundations are crucial to the ongoing creation, gathering, and validation of data.

The reason for starting the development of xAI models was the recognition that artificial intelligence models are often described as "black boxes," meaning that neither engineers nor users of the model can completely explain or comprehend how the algorithm arrives at predictions and recommendations in a particular health procedure. xAI enhances current AI technologies by highlighting application

---

L. Poslon (✉) · A. Čartolovni
Digital Healthcare Ethics Laboratory (Digit-HeaL), Catholic University of Croatia, Zagreb, Croatia
e-mail: luka.poslon@unicath.hr; anto.cartolovni@unicath.hr

R. Ortale et al. (eds.), *Explainable Machine Intelligence in Healthcare*,
https://doi.org/10.1007/978-3-031-91379-2_3

process flaws with the use of easy-to-interpret tools like heatmaps, saliency maps, decision rules, decision trees, and scatter plots.

In this chapter, we will analyze application examples of xAI tools and techniques which already exist and are used in healthcare such as Transparency and Interpretability For Understandability (TIFU) framework and others. To fully realize the promise of AI applications in healthcare, we would like to propose a new method for developing measurements for explanations inside the decision-making process, based on the work of existing frameworks. In addition to lowering bias and strengthening the patient-physician relationship, this approach should restore trust in the use of AI in healthcare. Additionally, this approach requires considering legal and regulatory compliance with laws and regulations including the Chinese PIPL, the American HIPAA, and the European GDPR.

Keywords xAI · Decision-making process · Healthcare · Medical AI · Trust · Enhancing trust · Interpretability · UQ · AI limits

1 Introduction

Predictions coming from AI are not always transparent to patients or physicians. Particularly in the context of healthcare high-risk scenarios, it is extremely important to know how AI models get to predictions, and explainability and transparency should be the primary focus of future research initiatives. Some may argue that there is nothing specifically new in AI when it comes to decision-making process, since humans also make decisions that are nontransparent, and physicians already employ computationally complicated models in their research and are adept at adjusting to AI advancements. Also, physicians already give patients insightful action suggestions while also using algorithmic decision support tools [1].

But there is a key distinction between the models that are now in use and other models: ML models are opaque [2], which is why people find them extremely difficult to comprehend the logic behind the model's predictions. The "decision-making" part of the model is difficult to translate to ideas that are easily understood by people. According to Zednik, the conventional wisdom in the nascent area of explainable artificial intelligence (xAI) is that opacity has to be decreased [3].

One of the key areas for improvement is the complex interrelationship that emerges while making decisions in the healthcare setting [4]. During the decision-making process, post hoc explanations combined with an AI system that has been prospectively verified and retrospectively assessed can help meet patients' and physicians' explanatory demands in the context of AI-supported medical decision-making.

Lack of opacity creates challenges regarding the trust that physicians and patients would place in AI systems since they are starting to be adopted in real-life contexts.

Also, working with "black box" models raises important ethical issues like informed consent. The creation of the xAI model increases the model's transparency and provides an explanation for algorithmic process prediction, which is essential for patients and healthcare professionals to gain trust in the use of AI in healthcare. For patients and healthcare professionals to be able to comprehend and believe the model's predictions and suggestions, it is imperative that AI models be transparently explained to them. This will also help ensure that the technology is widely used in clinical settings. For many years, obtaining a patient's informed consent in medicine required filling out a paper form that included details on the procedure they would be undergoing as well as the advantages and disadvantages of taking part in research. More and more information are being gathered online and kept in massive datasets that will be accessed by several academics and organizations for a variety of purposes in the future as a result of the advancement of digital healthcare technology and the incorporation of medical AI applications. In numerous clinical processes where processing times are measured in seconds, clinicians benefit from the incorporation of medical AI applications in decision-making process. When it comes to making medical diagnoses, disease prognoses, or treatment suggestions, physicians particularly like to rely on AI systems. Even AI assistance in terms of decision support technologies could improve physicians' cognitive and analytical skills; physicians should bear most responsibility for diagnoses, disease prognoses, or treatment suggestions and should do everything in their power to enable informed decisions for the patient. That responsibility involves complex interactions with an AI model in order to identify patterns in data and produce predictions. However, there are benefits as well as ethical risks and difficulties associated with using artificial intelligence in clinical decision-making or practice.

An early example of a computer program named "Advice Taker," which was presented by McCarthy in 1958 as a "program with common sense," shows that there was a connection between the explainable possibilities and AI development from the outset [5]. It is one of the first attempts suggesting that the secret to comprehending AI is having common sense talents. Even so, a few decades after that endeavor, there are still insufficiently precise guidelines and standards for the transparency and explainability of AI models, which would allow us to comply with the moral requirements of informed consent in medical practice. Explainability, a crucial component in high-risk medical decision-making, should offer a sufficient degree of comprehensibility for the average individual to enhance safety and win patient trust, even as the transparency of the AI model should aid in the quest for a direct understanding of the mechanism by which the AI model functions. In contrast to merely resolving problems with pattern recognition, recent research has placed an increasing emphasis on how AI systems should be able to construct a picture of the world that supports explanation and understanding [6].

1.1 The Challenges of Implementing AI in Healthcare

There are challenges to the broad use of AI in healthcare. Human or AI errors, among other causes, might cause these challenges. Human error may be one of these causes, especially if we make mistakes in specifying the objective, which the algorithm manages to accomplish despite not being our primary goal. AI has been prone to errors in various scenarios, including when training data was poor quality and models failed to comprehend the complete context of image recognition or autonomous operation. Image recognition and autonomous operation are crucial for healthcare and medicine since they are necessary for diagnosis or treatment recommendations. AI systems may be constantly improved by solving these issues with xAI, ensuring adequate training data, and assuring contextual comprehension.

Rapid technological advancements in the healthcare industry are producing massive amounts of data in different health databases, necessitating the optimization of patient care and the use of medical resources and the transition from manual to automated healthcare systems [7]. Utilizing contemporary technology like artificial intelligence—which has garnered significant attention for its ability to forecast unfavorable health outcomes for high-risk groups and provide prerequisites for public health interventions—is one way to address the issues posed by automation [8].

In time-sensitive medical situations, AI algorithms can swiftly and accurately make predictions based on high-dimensional data—a feat that humans may never be able to do either physically or mentally. Physicians might more accurately interpret the results based on reasoning and past knowledge if we could explain the many choices made by a given model and the precise features examined to obtain a certain conclusion.

The use of AI in healthcare is fraught with technological, ethical, legal, and sociological issues, all of which are listed in various studies, the majority of which are devoted to examining the fundamental ideas, obstacles, or real-world uses of AI [9, 10]. Some of the most important challenges are related to trust [11], explainability, transparency, opacity [12], bias, and fairness [13].

And while the concepts of fairness and transparency have a lot to do with how we provide information, how we use AI, and what we include in the design of the process itself, bias may cause an algorithm to fail to recognize important connections between input and output. Algorithms that are biased are less able to represent real relationships and true predictions.

Some authors were trying to answer the question: Could transparency be a sufficient solution to the opacity of LLM systems used in medicine [14]? We believe that transparency alone will not address the issues of utilizing opaque AI models in healthcare when the core logic is opaque to human examination. Understanding and having control over something do not necessarily follow from seeing it. The pursuit of transparency can be harmful and fail to give patients and physicians the information they need to put their faith in the system or hold the decision-maker responsible. Opacity in AI models raises concerns when clinicians must explain things to patients and when diagnosis and therapy must be supported by evidence. That is why we see explainability and xAI as expanded solution of transparency, which could help us in solving and minimizing the opacity in AI models.

It is not simple to achieve explainability and ensure proper explanation in the framework of healthcare. Researchers agree that the application of AI models on real-life scenarios asks for implementation of additional safeguards, while it is possible for AI models to amplify biases or cause prediction failures [15]. The lack of explanations or references makes it difficult to determine the validity and reliability of the information provided.

Current talks on technological possibilities of explainability mostly include two viewpoints: xAI and interpretable models. The goal of xAI is to create algorithms that can post-hoc explain specific characteristics of the black box model [16]. The use of AI models that are naturally comprehensible by humans and hence not opaque is referred to as using interpretable models, albeit there may be a trade-off in accuracy [17].

However, as explainability is important in the clinical setting from the standpoint of a physician, we shall concentrate on explainability-related situations. Due to this, Tom Miller [18] and Bertram Malle [19] argue that we should teach algorithms how to become explainable, which has a twofold meaning: to find meaning for algorithmic decisions and govern social connections. Finding meaning includes resolving conflicts or inconsistencies in our knowledge systems, which frequently arise from discrepancies between our understanding and the state of the outside world. Creating shared meanings, changing views, or swaying behavior are all components of governing social interaction. Understanding AI predictions is vital in their clinician's daily life, and specialized fields such as healthcare are prepared and trained to deal with high-level patient risk [20]. Considering that xAI techniques can reduce the opacity of the algorithm hiding behind a "black box," we might identify and decrease the incidence of aleatoric and epistemic uncertainty using xAI methods. AI applications in healthcare dealing with uncertainties could only become increasingly effective with the help of xAI methods. The area of explainable AI serves a purpose and is essential and offers a significant possibility for AI solutions in healthcare. Explainability allows one to identify doubts or to explain how they came to be without depending on which side of a discussion one is on with an AI system or human experts.

xAI aims to illuminate an AI system's capacity for explaining its decision-making process. It aids in our better comprehension of how underlying predictions are formed. As a result, xAI may increase trust in the use of AI in healthcare and how we employ AI models, leading to a broader social acceptance of these technologies.

xAI can make algorithmic predictions in its interpretations more intuitive for humans, improve therapeutic relationships, and foster trust in implementations of AI in healthcare. But besides interpretations, xAI methods in biomedicine are also useful for optimization of the models used in radiology or dermatology through saliency maps [21]. In addition, xAI methods can enhance both the precision and the cost-effectiveness of AI models by incorporating cost-aware analyses [22]. An additional advantage is offered by frameworks such as EXPRESS (explainable predictions for gene expression data) which not only explain why specific combination of drugs in cancer therapy may have a synergistic effect, but also uidentify the genes associated with that synergy. Together, these insights can significantly improve the efficacy of medical procedures [23].

The use of supercomputing in biomedical simulations potentially revolutionizes healthcare, enabling unprecedented advances in disease modeling, drug discovery, cancer care, and personalized medicine [24]. However, the field faces significant ethical challenges and regulatory obstacles with AI-enabled supercomputing that must be addressed to ensure responsible innovation. The chapter delves into the complex boundary conditions in healthcare simulations, highlighting the need for robust ethical frameworks and adaptive regulatory mechanisms to address data requirements, privacy concerns, and potential biases while also highlighting the regulatory landscape's discrepancies. Since there are currently no internationally standardized rules or regulations pertaining to the use of AI in medicine that would standardize the conduct of physicians, further research and development in this field are required [25].

1.2 xAI Methods for Ensuring Trust and Transparency

There is a trend showing that xAI is starting to be more and more important in medicine and healthcare [26]. AI models such as XGBoost [27], which can predict the functional status of kidney pre-transplant—an important predictor of post-transplant survival—could be combined with methods of xAI (e.g., SHAP) to provide interpretable predictions, helping clinicians and patients understand and potentially trust the model outputs.

xAI can make algorithmic predictions more intuitive for human users, improve therapeutic relationship, and build trust in the implementation of AI in healthcare [28]. Reducing the opacity of black box AI systems is crucial for healthcare AI applications because of the moral and professional responsibility of physicians to provide reasons and explanations for their decisions [29]. Also, with this strategy, patients are guaranteed to get therapies that are especially matched to their unique requirements, improving their quality of life and resulting in better outcomes. There is thus a justifiable worry about relying on the algorithmic predictions since it might well lead to misdiagnosis or false prognosis. As such, the explanation needed is one which provides grounds for relying on the system's output—for trusting the system as a useful tool in the medical context.

AI tools in healthcare provides support by improving evidence-based decision-making and efficiency, enhancing diagnostics, speed, and the delivery of prognosis or treatment for patients. Those advancements helped a lot with creating personalized treatment plans and building patient trust in the implementation of AI in healthcare. The healthcare sector's constant focus is finding the ideal balance between finding potential benefits and possible threats associated with technological revolution.

Achieving AI systems that are trustworthy for all stakeholders in th ehealthcare sector is a challenging task, as trustworthiness is a multifaceted concept encompassing a range of cognitive, emotional, and behavioral components [30]. Even when physicans lack full knowledge or understanding of drug pharmacology, studies have shown that patients are often willing to use drugs that are demonstrably safe and effective, highlighting that trust can exist based on evidence of safety and efficacy rather than complete understanding by all intermediaries [31].

Trust as a cornerstone of every human relationship should be the base for developing healthcare sector, which patients would comprehend is organized in such a way that the least possible mistakes could happen over the course of treatment [31].

Black box models in AI are generally thought to pose a problem for trustworthiness. For example, despite the fact that robotic surgical systems are as efficient as a physician, many patients still trust a surgeon more than a robotic system [32]. According to several authors, the lack of model interpretability causes a decrease of trust in current diagnostic models, particularly regarding the use of xAI in breast cancer applications [33]. Methods of xAI could help with providing explanations for generated predictions enabling patients to assess the trustworthiness of the underlying black box model [34].

1.3 Enhancing Trustworthiness with xAI

Including transparency at multiple points of development, test, and implementation stages of medical AI [35] can move medical AI toward fairness and reduce bias. If we make using medical AI more transparent, it will be easier to recognize and remove bias. The concepts of fairness and transparency have a lot to do with how we provide information, how we use AI, and what we include in the design of the process itself. Transparency is one of the most widely discussed principles in the AI ethics debate and is becoming one of the defining characteristics and can be defined as "the search for a direct understanding of the mechanism by which a model works"[36].

Transparency of fair AI algorithms is crucial for the concept of trust. It is of utmost importance to work toward fair medical AI so that physicians and patients can regain trust in medical AI.

Trust in medical AI can be regained by adequately approaching the concept of fairness and not just looking at the algorithm as a mathematical construct but by observing how algorithm works in practice and how it affects the real world.

1.4 UQ for Enhancing Trustworthiness

Many case studies remind us how important it is to question algorithmic predictions [37]. To say that one AI system is trustworthy is more than to say that one can rely on that AI system. Reliability is insufficient to generate trustworthiness [38]. But understanding how and why an algorithm came to particular prediction is not just a problem of computer science, but the need for fair and just predictions are related to the possibility of understanding AI. Therefore, epistemology and ethics play a central role [39].

This discussion explores limitations of trust and explainability in healthcare scenarios during the decision-making processes [40]. Particularly, we concentrate on limitations which are showing when uncertainty quantification (UQ) in healthcare scenario is present and discuss how quantification of uncertainties is helping to build trust in AI systems. According to Grote, the possibility of overreliance on AI could be decreased if physicians are appropriately informed about the risk of model uncertainty with uncertainty quantification during the medical diagnosis process [41]. It is imperative to provide time abstention in cases where UQ indicates that physicians should take a second look at the patient [42]. This could be used as a safety measure and help building trust. Other authors claim that UQ can improve reliability of model predictions even in scenarios involving missing or noisy data [43].

Our work discusses the limitations of UQ in line with research by Guotai Wang [44], Jakob Gawlikowski [45], Jeroen Vranken [46], and Zhibin Liao [47]. But AI systems without UQ assessment tools cannot differentiate between aleatoric and epistemic uncertainty and thus might fail to improve model accuracy at all [48].

Still, there are many challenges associated with UQ: absence of theory, absence of causal models, sensitivity to imperfect data, and computational feasibility [49]. There are also different approaches which address challenges associated with UQ and increasing trustworthiness. Wang et al. suggest improving aleatoric uncertainty by longer test time [44]. Vranek et al. showed in their analyses of ECG classification that the accuracy of models increased when estimated uncertain samples were removed [46]. Gawlikowski et al. mention safety challenges if explainability is missing [45]. It was shown by Ghali et al. that more run time and memory are required for better predicting combined uncertainties. These findings have a significant impact on the trustworthiness of AI systems and provide valuable insights into how to enhance the data utilized to make better predictions [50].

Clearly understanding, measuring, and assessing uncertainties are vital for enhancing trust. UQ done right could therefore improve patient care, build trust, and provide more accurate predictions. We critique existing AI systems that lack QU assessment tools. We suggest these systems will ultimately fail to fulfill desired explainability and transparency criteria, which will prevent their adoption in the healthcare context.

1.5 Chinese PIPL, US HIPAA, and European GDPR

There have been different initiatives in various countries to implement policies and legislation. Three main legal frameworks that aim to protect people's data privacy are the European General Data Protection Regulation (GDPR), the United States Health Insurance Portability and Accountability Act (HIPAA), and the Chinese Personal Information Protection Law (PIPL). However, their goals and areas of application differ greatly. China's comprehensive data protection legislation, known as PIPL, places a strong emphasis on state control and national security while regulating the gathering, using, and sharing of personal data in all spheres of society. HIPAA, on the other hand, is unique to the healthcare sector in the United States and focuses on protecting patient privacy and medical records while allowing data interchange across the healthcare system [51].

A complete set of regulations for guaranteeing the confidentiality and security of health information is provided by the HIPAA [52], while one of the most extensive and strict privacy rules is GDPR, which has an influence on how businesses manage the data of EU people everywhere [53].

Regarding the extent and type of data they safeguard, the GDPR and HIPAA reflect two distinct approaches to data protection. The former uses a thorough strategy that is applicable to both organizations that gather and process personal data as well as personal data itself. In contrast, the USA now uses a sector-specific strategy to safeguard personal information, relying on a disjointed mix of federal and state rules, regulations, common law torts, and constitutional protections [53].

The GDPR's extraterritorial scope is another significant distinction. In contrast to HIPAA, the GDPR is applicable to entities that gather or handle personal data of persons within the European Economic Area (EEA), irrespective of the entity's actual location inside the EEA's member nations [54]. On the other hand, HIPAA does not specifically provide for extraterritorial reach, the federal Department of Health and Human Services (HSS) has not yet pursued enforcement action against a foreign organization found in violation of the law [55].

Although the PIPL shares many characteristics with the GDPR, the underlying forces influencing China's legislative trajectory are neither simple and one-dimensional. Pragmatic legal growth was illustrated by China's willingness to experiment with sectors like cybersecurity, criminal law, and consumer protection. The choice to experiment and modify several legal tools rather than jumping right into a single, all-encompassing data protection framework was both in line with China's legal culture and indicative of the proposal's initial intent [56].

Here we will try to show the major differences between Chinese PIPL, US HIPAA, and European GDPR.

Major differences			
	GDPR	HIPAA	PIPL
Accountability	Accountability premise expressed clearly	Accountability premise expressed clearly	Accountability premise expressed clearly
Sensitive personal data	Sensitive personal data handling must have specific justification. Allows people to request that an institution delete their data, a right known as the right to be forgotten	Medical records and other personal information cannot be altered or deleted (the information is stored forever)	Sensitive personal data processing requires separate written approval
Consent	Justification for handling personal data in a permissible manner. High quality if it can be trusted	The consent form must be accompanied by a privacy notice. HIPAA consent must be separate from the normal informed consent for treatment. The consent must be in plain language and signed by the patient. The patient may revoke that consent at any time	A valid legal foundation for processing personal data in a legitimate manner (permission or statutory consent free scenarios). Under the PIPL, legitimate interest is not a legitimate foundation
Data export	Data processors are directly obligated	Requires that all parties involved are responsible for protecting the data. This includes health organizations like hospitals, clinics, and insurance as well as companies like Dropbox or cloud service providers	The sole notion of a data handler, with no legal distinction made between a data controller and a data processor
Sanctions	Data protection authorities can impose administrative fines. Data subjects can bring civil actions for compensation	Depending on the degree of responsibility, civil monetary penalties for HIPAA infractions can range from $137 to $68,928 per infraction. Intentional infractions may also result in criminal sanctions, which include fines and sometimes even jail time	Administrative punishment: fines on personal data handler, warning, confiscation of illegal gains, suspension or termination of operation, public disclosure of noncompliance

1.6 Algorithmic Fairness Enhancing Trust in AI

As medical AI is used to improve healthcare quality and efficiency and to alleviate challenges related to a growing number of patients facing a lack of physicians, it is increasingly involved in decision-making processes.

Algorithmic fairness is an area at the intersection of machine learning and ethics with the main goal of embedding fairness and equity into the algorithm and evaluating existing biases in data. Algorithm fairness is investigating causes of unfairness, measurements of fairness, building fair algorithms, and regulating machine learning. Training a "fair" predictive algorithm is an optimization task among "fair" solutions defined by hard constraints. It is no longer important that the model should exhibit accuracy, efficiency, or profitability; it should also be fair.

In the public space, one can hear how algorithms in the decision-making process can be used as tools to enforce equality due to the algorithmic ability to overcome cognitive limitations and social biases that arise from human nature. It is hoped that this enables more objective and fair decisions [57]. But challenges of algorithmic fairness are widespread, and they are not reserved only to the application of AI in medicine. We can also find cases in other human activities such as the criminal justice system. AI algorithms developed for the criminal justice system in the United States of America classified African American defendants who did not reoffend as high risk at a significantly higher rate than white defendants who did not reoffend. The prediction was made based on historical arrest records [58].

The approach to algorithm fairness does not include just quantitative methods because reasons for fairness go beyond just algorithm and data.

Exploring the field of algorithm fairness can make us aware that imperfect data can lead to the wrong path but also that algorithms themselves are not value-neutral, while algorithmic decision-making systems incorporate the values and preferences of particular stakeholders which are in line with the prediction of an algorithm. Reasons for unfairness can be many: historical bias, a bias that stems from the algorithmic objectives, an unbalanced dataset, missing data or values, algorithm opacity, or proxy variables. This technical limitation makes a central question about algorithmic fairness: How can physicians support equitable decisions with algorithms?

1.7 TIFU (Transparency and Interpretability for Understandability) Framework in Healthcare

The growing prevalence of medical AI in clinical settings begs the moral dilemma of what level of explainability is necessary for the ethical and appropriate usage of AI-based solutions in medical settings [59]. Assessment tools on which we are developing double standards should be carefully examined before the practical implementation in healthcare.

Opaque AI systems have to be viewed as preprocessing modules, and simpler interpretable models with transparent outputs and interpretable downstream classification tasks should be suggested for model usage.

The three major focuses of the TIFU framework are (a) computational structures and processes, (b) output display, and (c) how inputs and data connect to the clinical domain [60]. Although the TIFU framework does not ensure explainability in the full sense, development is based on the principles in the general xAI literature, extending these principles to specific considerations for psychiatry and mental health, which could be interesting direction for further development of decision-making applications. The goal of the TIFU framework is to increase the precision and coherence of explainability, and results could be useful for other similar applications.

2 Conclusion

If we design medical AI well, it may provide a way to audit and improve the way care is being delivered to patients. AI medical fairness is not just about preventing a model from harming a protected group, it may also help focus care where it is needed.

Despite AI's potential, human oversight remains critical due to the variability in users' expertise and the complex nature of AI predictions. Trustworthy data and adherence to explainability and transparency standards are essential for the ethical and legal application of AI. The development of xAI models addresses the "black box" nature of traditional AI by providing interpretable tools like heatmaps and decision trees.

We suggest that AI models used in healthcare, such as XGBoost (which can be combined with explainable AI methods like SHAP) or other xAI frameworks like TIFU, can provide interpretable predictions that help clinicians and patients understand both the underlying mechanisms of the models and the relative importance of individual predictions in the clinical decision-making process.

We have to look at the real-world impact and what is happening in practice because just relying on the mathematical notion of fairness does not lead to deeper equality and fairness in medical AI.

References

1. Freiesleben, T. What does explainable AI explain? Dissertation, LMU München: Graduate School of Systemic Neurosciences (GSN). 2023
2. Sullivan E. Understanding from machine learning models. Br J Philos Sci. 2022;73(1):109–33. https://doi.org/10.1093/bjps/axz035.
3. Zednik C. Solving the black box problem: a normative framework for explainable artificial intelligence. Philos Technol. 2021;34(2):265–88.

4. O'Hara K. Explainable AI and the philosophy and practice of explanation. Compu Law Secur Rev. 2020;39:105474. https://doi.org/10.1016/j.clsr.2020.105474.
5. McCarthy, J. Programs with common sense. Paper presented at the meeting of the proceedings of the Teddington conference on the mechanization of thought processes, London, 1959.
6. Lake BM, Ullman TD, Tenenbaum JB, Gershman SJ. Building machines that learn and think like people. Behav Brain Sci. 2017;40:e253. https://doi.org/10.1017/S0140525X16001837.
7. Wubineh BZ, Deriba FG, Woldeyohannis MM. Exploring the opportunities and challenges of implementing artificial intelligence in healthcare: a systematic literature review. Urol Oncol. 2024;42(3):48–56. https://doi.org/10.1016/j.urolonc.2023.11.019.
8. Chen M, Decary M. Artificial intelligence in healthcare: an essential guide for health leaders. Healthc Manage Forum. 2020;33(1):10–8. https://doi.org/10.1177/0840470419873123.
9. Giansanti D, Di Basilio F. The artificial intelligence in digital radiology: part 1: the challenges, acceptance and consensus. Healthcare (Basel, Switzerland). 2022;10(3):509. https://doi.org/10.3390/healthcare10030509.
10. Ashton JJ, Young A, Johnson MJ, et al. Using machine learning to impact on long-term clinical care: principles, challenges, and practicalities. Pediatr Res. 2023;93:324–33. https://doi.org/10.1038/s41390-022-02194-6.
11. Jeyaraman M, Balaji S, Jeyaraman N, Yadav S. Unraveling the ethical enigma: artificial intelligence in healthcare. Cureus. 2023;15(8):e43262. https://doi.org/10.7759/cureus.43262.
12. Balasubramaniam N, Kauppinen M, Hiekkanen K, Kujala S. Transparency and explainability of AI systems: ethical guidelines in practice. In: Gervasi V, Vogelsang A, editors. Requirements engineering: foundation for software quality. REFSQ 2022, Lecture notes in computer science, vol. 13216. Cham: Springer; 2022. https://doi.org/10.1007/978-3-030-98464-9_1.
13. Ferrara E. Fairness and bias in artificial intelligence: a brief survey of sources, impacts, and mitigation strategies. Science. 2024;6(1):3. https://doi.org/10.3390/sci6010003.
14. Lexchin J, Fugh-Berman A. A ray of sunshine: transparency in physician-industry relationships is not enough. J Gen Intern Med. 2021;36(10):3194–8. https://doi.org/10.1007/s11606-021-06657-0.
15. Banerjee I, Bhattacharjee K, Burns JL, Trivedi H, Purkayastha S, Seyyed-Kalantari L, Patel BN, Shiradkar R, Gichoya J. "Shortcuts" causing bias in radiology artificial intelligence: causes, evaluation, and mitigation. J Am Coll Radiol. 2023;20(9):842–51. https://doi.org/10.1016/j.jacr.2023.06.025.
16. Ordish J, Brigden T, Hall A. Black box medicine and transparency: the ethics of transparency and explanation. PHG Foundation. 2020.; https://www.phgfoundation.org/documents/black-box-ethics-transparency-explanation.pdf
17. Rudin C. Stop explaining black box machine learning models for high stakes decisions and use interpretable models instead. Nat Mach Intell. 2019;1:206–15.
18. Miller T. Explanation in artificial intelligence: insights from the social sciences. In: CoRR abs/1706.07269; 2017. arXiv: 1706.07269. http:arxiv.org/abs/1706.07269.
19. Malle B. How the mind explains behavior: folk explanation, meaning and social interaction. MIT Press; 2004.
20. Gerdes A. The role of explainability in AI-supported medical decision-making. Discov Artif Intell. 2024;4:29. https://doi.org/10.1007/s44163-024-00119-2.
21. DeGrave AJ, Janizek JD, Lee SI. AI for radiographic COVID-19 detection selects shortcuts over signal. medRxiv: the preprint server for health sciences, 2020.09.13.20193565. 2020; https://doi.org/10.1101/2020.09.13.20193565.
22. Erion G, Janizek JD, Hudelson C, Utarnachitt RB, McCoy AM, Sayre MR, White NJ, Lee SI. A cost-aware framework for the development of AI models for healthcare applications. Nat Biomed Eng. 2022;6(12):1384–98. https://doi.org/10.1038/s41551-022-00872-8.
23. Janizek JD, Dincer AB, Celik S, Chen H, Chen W, Naxerova K, Lee SI. Uncovering expression signatures of synergistic drug responses via ensembles of explainable machine-learning models. Nat Biomed Eng. 2023;7(6):811–29. https://doi.org/10.1038/s41551-023-01034-0.
24. Ross C, Swetlitz I. IBM pitched its Watson supercomputer as a revolution in cancer care. It's nowhere close. 2017. https://www.statnews.com/2017/09/05/watson-ibm-cancer/

25. Jiang L, Wu Z, Xu X, Zhan Y, Jin X, Wang L, Qiu Y. Opportunities and challenges of artificial intelligence in the medical field: current application, emerging problems, and problem-solving strategies. J Int Med Res. 2021;49(3):3000605211000157. https://doi.org/10.1177/03000605211000157.
26. Hulsen T. Explainable artificial intelligence (XAI): concepts and challenges in healthcare. AI. 2023;4:652–66. https://doi.org/10.3390/ai4030034.
27. Mark E, Goldsman D, Gurbaxani B, Keskinocak P, Sokol J. Predicting a kidney transplant patient's pre-transplant functional status based on information from waitlist registration. Sci Rep. 2023;13(1):6164. https://doi.org/10.1038/s41598-023-33117-y.
28. Nasarian E, Alizadehsani R, Acharya U, Tsui K-L. Designing interpretable ML system to enhance Trust in Healthcare: a systematic review to proposed responsible clinician-AI-collaboration framework. Inf Fusion. 2024;108:102412. https://doi.org/10.1016/j.inffus.2024.102412.
29. Holzinger A, Biemann C, Pattichis C, Kell D. What do we need to build explainable AI systems for the medical domain? 2017. https://arxiv.org/1712.09923
30. Boddington P. Towards a code of ethics for artificial intelligence (artificial intelligence: foundations, theory, and algorithms). 1st ed. Springer; 2017.
31. Palmer SW. The role of trust in facilitating human-AI relationships. 2024.
32. Longoni C, Bonezzi A, Morewedge CK. Resistance to medical artificial intelligence. J Consum Res. 2019;46(4):629–50. https://doi.org/10.1093/jcr/ucz013.
33. Bidwai P, Khairnar S, Gite S. Explainable artificial intelligence in breast cancer identification. In: Explainable AI in healthcare. Chapman and Hall/CRC; 2023. p. 148–65. https://doi.org/10.1201/9781003333425-8.
34. Band SS, Yarahmadi A, Hsu CC, Biyari M, Sookhak M, Ameri R, Dehzangi I, Chronopoulos AT, Liang HW. Application of explainable artificial intelligence in medical health: a systematic review of interpretability methods. Inf Med Unlocked. 2023;40:101286. https://doi.org/10.1016/j.imu.2023.101286.
35. Mccradden MD, Joshi S, Mazwi M, Anderson JA. Ethical limitations of algorithmic fairness solutions in health care machine learning. Lancet Digit Health. 2020;2:e221–3. https://doi.org/10.1016/s2589-7500(20)30065-0.
36. Akinci D'Antonoli T. Ethical considerations for artificial intelligence: an overview of the current radiology landscape. Diagn Interv Imaging. 2020;26:504–11. https://doi.org/10.5152/dir.2020.19279.
37. Gaube S, Suresh H, Raue M, Merritt A, Berkowitz SJ, Lermer E, Coughlin JF, Guttag JV, Colak E, Ghassemi M. Do as AI say: susceptibility in deployment of clinical decision-aids. NPJ Digit Med. 2021;4(31):1–8. https://doi.org/10.1038/s41746-021-00385-9.
38. Hatherley JJ. Limits of trust in medical AI. J Med Ethics. 2020;46(7):478–81. https://doi.org/10.1136/medethics-2019-105935.
39. Russo F, Schliesser E, Wagemans J. Connecting ethics and epistemology of AI. AI & Soc. 2023;39:1585. https://doi.org/10.1007/s00146-022-01617-6.
40. Quinn TP, Senadeera M, Jacobs S, Coghlan S, Le V. Trust and medical AI: the challenges we face and the expertise needed to overcome them. J Am Med Inform Assoc. 2021;28(4):890–4. https://doi.org/10.1093/jamia/ocaa268.
41. Grote T. Trustworthy medical AI systems need to know when they don't know. J Med Ethics. 2021;47:337–8.
42. Kompa B, Snoek J, Beam AL. Second opinion needed: communicating uncertainty in medical machine learning. NPJ Digit Med. 2021;4, 4:4. https://doi.org/10.1038/s41746-020-00367-3.
43. Seoni S, Jahmunah V, Salvi M, Barua PD, Molinari F, Acharya UR. Application of uncertainty quantification to artificial intelligence in healthcare: a review of last decade (2013–2023). Comput Biol Med. 2023;165:107441. https://doi.org/10.1016/j.compbiomed.2023.107441.
44. Wang G, Li W, Aertsen M, Deprest J, Ourselin S, Vercauteren T. Aleatoric uncertainty estimation with test-time augmentation for medical image segmentation with convolutional neural networks. Neurocomputing. 2019;338:34–45. https://doi.org/10.1016/j.neucom.2019.01.103.

45. Gawlikowski J, Tassi CRN, Ali M, et al. A survey of uncertainty in deep neural networks. Artif Intell Rev. 2023;56(Suppl 1):1513–89. https://doi.org/10.1007/s10462-023-10562-9.
46. Vranken JF, van de Leur RR, Gupta DK, Orozco LEJ, Hassink RJ, van der Harst P, Doevendans PA, Gulshad S, van Es R. Uncertainty estimation for deep learning-based automated analysis of 12-lead electrocardiograms. Eur Heart J Digit Health. 2021;2(3):401–15. https://doi.org/10.1093/ehjdh/ztab045.
47. Liao Z, et al. On modelling label uncertainty in deep neural networks: automatic estimation of intra- observer variability in 2D echocardiography quality assessment. IEEE Trans Med Imaging. 2019;39:1868–83.
48. Yu J, Wang D, Zheng M. Uncertainty quantification: can we trust artificial intelligence in drug discovery? iScience. 2022;25(8):104814. https://doi.org/10.1016/j.isci.2022.104814.
49. Begoli E, Bhattacharya T, Kusnezov D. The need for uncertainty quantification in machine-assisted medical decision making. Nature. 2019;1:20. https://doi.org/10.1038/s42256-018-0004-1.
50. Ghali H, Yoon S, Won D. Uncertainty quantification for healthcare data. In: IISE annual conference. Proceedings. Institute of Industrial and Systems Engineers (IISE); 2023. p. 1–7. https://doi.org/10.13140/RG.2.2.14608.99847.
51. Shojaei P, Vlahu-Gjorgievska E, Chow Y-W. Security and privacy of technologies in health information systems: a systematic literature review. Computers. 2024;13(2):41. https://doi.org/10.3390/computers13020041.
52. Mbonihankuye S, Nkunzimana A, Ndagijimana A. Healthcare data security technology: HIPAA compliance. Wirel Commun Mob Comput. 2019;2019:1927495.
53. Fathima Shah W. Preserving privacy and security: a comparative study of health data regulations – GDPR vs. HIPAA. Int J Res Appl Sci Eng Technol. 2023;11:11.
54. Bradford L, Aboy M, Liddell K. International transfers of health data between the EU and USA: a sector-specific approach for the USA to ensure an 'adequate' level of protection. J Law Biosci. 2020;7(1):lsaa055. https://doi.org/10.1093/jlb/lsaa055.
55. Tovino SA. The HIPAA privacy rule and the EU GDPR: illustrative comparisons. Seton Hall Law Rev. 2017;47(4):973–93.
56. Li W, Chen J. From Brussels effect to gravity assists: understanding the evolution of the GDPR-inspired personal information protection law in China. Comput Law Secur Rev. 2024;54:105994.
57. Green B. Escaping the impossibility of fairness: from formal to Substan-tive algorithmic fairness. Philos Technol. 2022;35 https://doi.org/10.1007/s13347-022-00584-6.
58. Kleinberg J. Inherent trade-offs in algorithmic fairness. SIGMETRICS perform. Eval Rev. 2018;46(1):40. https://doi.org/10.1145/3292040.3219634.
59. Kempt H, Heilinger JC, Nagel SK. Relative explainability and double standards in medical decision-making. Ethics Inf Technol. 2022;24:20. https://doi.org/10.1007/s10676-022-09646-x.
60. Joyce DW, Kormilitzin A, Smith KA, et al. Explainable artificial intelligence for mental health through transparency and interpretability for understandability. NPJ Digit Med. 2023;6, 6:6. https://doi.org/10.1038/s41746-023-00751-9.

Shedding Light Inside the Black Box: Techniques for Explainable Artificial Intelligence in Healthcare

Loris Belcastro, Riccardo Cantini, Fabrizio Marozzo, Domenico Talia, and Paolo Trunfio

Contents

Abstract Artificial intelligence techniques and systems are demonstrating their effectiveness in solving problems in many application areas, including healthcare. Over the years, several studies focused on leveraging machine learning and deep learning techniques to identify diseases in patients. However, while these techniques have demonstrated remarkable accuracy in diagnosis, they often operate as "black-box" models, meaning they provide outputs without clear explanations of the rationale behind their decisions. This lack of transparency poses significant challenges, particularly in the healthcare domain, where decisions can have significant implications for the well-being of patients and treatment paths. In response to this challenge, explainable artificial intelligence (XAI) has emerged as a research area aiming at providing not only accurate diagnoses but also understandable and interpretable explanations for the decisions made by AI models. For providing explanations also large language models (LLMs) may be exploited. This chapter provides an overview of cutting-edge XAI techniques for healthcare applications, which hold the promise of enhancing trust, enabling clinicians to better understand and contextualize AI results, and ultimately improving patient care. Nevertheless, XAI techniques in this domain produce explanations in a form that is not always

L. Belcastro (✉) · R. Cantini · F. Marozzo · D. Talia · P. Trunfio
DIMES, University of Calabria, Rende, Italy
e-mail: lbelcastro@dimes.unical.it; rcantini@dimes.unical.it; fmarozzo@dimes.unical.it; talia@dimes.unical.it; trunfio@dimes.unical.it

R. Ortale et al. (eds.), *Explainable Machine Intelligence in Healthcare*,
https://doi.org/10.1007/978-3-031-91379-2_4

easily understandable by healthcare professionals. Current conversational AI can play a crucial role in bridging this gap by transforming model explanations into a human-readable format, making them more accessible to clinicians and users. The chapter also presents a case study addressing the critical issue of disease detection using social media data, demonstrating how the integration of LLMs with XAI techniques allows to enhance model interpretability, facilitating efficient communication between the AI system and healthcare professionals.

Keywords BERT · ChatGPT · Depression detection · Large Language Models · Mental disorder · NaturaL Language Processing · XAI

1 Introduction

In the domain of artificial intelligence (AI), algorithm explainability necessitates that machine learning methods and their decisions or outcomes are comprehensible to humans at an acceptable level. A lack of explainability can lead to opacity in the design, application, evaluation, and control of these algorithms. Consequently, algorithms influencing human lives must be continuously monitored, evaluated, and refined. Without this oversight, they risk perpetuating the values and biases inherent in their creation, thereby amplifying the negative impacts of their decisions.

Introduced in 2004 by Van Lent et al., the concept of explainable AI (XAI) was to describe the ability of a system to elucidate the behavior of AI-controlled agents in simulation games. Today, XAI represents a scientific field dedicated to developing and implementing AI systems that are understandable to humans [4]. Grasping how algorithms and computers function is often challenging, especially when dealing with complex systems like those used in aviation, autonomous vehicles, DNA analysis, or nuclear submarines. AI systems rank among the most intricate human inventions, capable of executing sophisticated tasks and producing complex results through computations that even experts may struggle to interpret. Historically, the focus has been on explaining AI outputs and decisions post-operation. Recently, the demand has shifted toward designing AI systems whose rationale, operations, and semantics are inherently comprehensible to users.

XAI encompasses methods and techniques that produce machine learning algorithms capable of being understood and trusted by humans, along with the results and decisions they yield. In contrast, "black-box" AI systems operate without offering insight into how their decisions are made. These systems often utilize machine learning on large datasets, mapping features to predefined classes to predict behaviors or events without justifying the process. This opacity not only obscures transparency but also introduces the risk of biases stemming from human errors or discrimination embedded in training data, potentially leading to unjust or erroneous conclusions.

Machine learning techniques are broadly categorized into *supervised* and *unsupervised* algorithms. Supervised learning requires human intervention to train

algorithms using labeled data, enhancing their explainability by employing predefined classes. However, this approach does not entirely eliminate the black-box problem. In contrast, unsupervised learning relies on unlabeled data, requiring algorithms to autonomously identify patterns, often with minimal or no human input. This autonomy can reduce explainability, necessitating careful attention to prevent opaque, nontransparent solutions.

Deep learning systems, particularly those utilizing artificial neural networks, further complicate explainability. These networks encode training examples in their connection matrices, extrapolating them to infer outcomes for unseen data. In such systems, the connection weights among neurons can span gigabytes or terabytes. Unlike traditional software systems where problematic code segments can be identified and fixed, neural networks provide no explicit algorithmic steps, but only large matrices of weights. This opacity makes understanding unexpected outputs and their origins highly challenging. Addressing this issue by developing transparent and interpretable deep learning systems is a crucial research priority.

XAI methodologies aim to enhance human understanding of machine learning models by addressing accuracy, fairness, transparency, and decision-making outcomes. As defined by the Defense Advanced Research Projects Agency (DARPA), XAI seeks to create explainable models without sacrificing learning performance while enabling users to appropriately trust and manage AI systems. Moreover, the European Union's GDPR mandates a "right of explanation," granting individuals access to "meaningful information about the logic involved" in automated decisions with legal or significant effects. Achieving this right requires robust technologies and processes to elucidate the logic of AI-based decision systems, particularly those utilizing black-box models. The recommendation on artificial intelligence by the Organisation for Economic Co-operation and Development (OECD) emphasizes transparency and explainability, urging stakeholders to "commit to responsible disclosure regarding AI systems."

A significant gap in machine learning lies in the absence of clear, human-readable explanations of model logic and potential biases. Closing this gap improves transparency, accountability, ethics, and safety. The "black-box explanation" approach addresses this by associating decisions with interpretable reasoning, facilitating the auditing of machine learning algorithms. Large language models (LLMs) can further aid by providing human-readable descriptions of the reasoning behind machine or deep learning decisions, fostering greater trust and usability.

2 XAI Approaches in Healthcare

Machine learning (ML) and deep learning (DL) techniques are drastically changing the healthcare field by improving the accuracy and efficiency of diagnostic and prognostic processes. Every day more and more advanced algorithms are proposed to analyze complex medical data, identify patterns, and provide insights that support clinicians in making decisions, often surpassing the capabilities of human

experts. For example, DL has shown remarkable performance in identifying skin diseases [32], detecting COVID-19 [6], diagnosing retinal diseases [21], and classifying various malignancies from pathological images [28, 31].

Many research studies on depression and mental disorders examine the link between language and mental health symptoms to detect issues like depression, suicidal thoughts, and various health conditions (including influenza, pregnancy, and eating disorders) [41]. As social media has become widely popular, a vast number of individuals express their feelings, ideas, and life experiences, generating immense quantities of digital data that reveal their viewpoints, emotions, political leanings, and psychological conditions [11, 56]. The volume, velocity, and heterogeneity of this data are such that it is not easy to process with traditional computational approaches, requiring advanced big data processing techniques [12, 52]. Although managing large datasets is challenging, their application is crucial across numerous disciplines, including healthcare. For instance, information from social media can indicate potential mental health issues or depressive symptoms in users, highlighting the importance of developing effective detection systems. Consequently, numerous machine learning and deep learning approaches have been introduced to automate the detection of mental health disorders [3, 25, 33]. Studies leveraging machine learning to identify depression through social media have employed algorithms such as support vector machines, random forest, as well as techniques based on affective lexicons [5, 7, 24, 46, 50].

Deep learning techniques have gradually surpassed traditional machine learning approaches in many fields, thanks to their capacity to automatically learn features with minimal manual effort. In the context of detecting mental disorders, several studies have applied deep neural networks to uncover indicators of mental health conditions from social media data. For example, Kerasiotis et al.[29] proposed a novel approach to detecting depression in social media posts by leveraging transformer-based models, specifically DistilBERT, in combination with auxiliary features such as metadata and linguistic markers, demonstrating improved classification accuracy through data augmentation and deep learning techniques. Sell et al. [49] explored the use of ensembles of BERT variants to improve depression detection from clinical interview transcripts. By comparing individual BERT models with various ensemble strategies, the authors demonstrated that ensembles improve classification performance and enhance robustness across different clinical interviews. Expanding on these efforts, Po'swiata and Perełkiewicz [44] compared various transformer-based models and found RoBERTa to be the top performer. They further improved this approach by fine-tuning a specialized language model, DepRoBERTa, pre-trained on Reddit posts discussing depressive symptoms. To further improve accuracy, they employed ensemble averaging, combining DepRoBERTa with a fine-tuned RoBERTa-large model.

Despite these advances, the integration of these technologies into clinical practice has been limited by different factors. A significant obstacle is the "black-box" nature of ML/DL models, which makes it difficult for healthcare professionals to trust and understand their decisions. This lack of transparency can hinder the acceptance and use of these technologies in real-world, critical healthcare

settings. To address this challenge, there is a growing need for explainable artificial intelligence (XAI) techniques to make the decision-making processes of ML/DL models more transparent and interpretable. By explaining the "how" and "why" behind model predictions, XAI can help clinicians understand and have confidence in these advanced technologies. This is especially important in healthcare, where understanding the reasons behind a classification result can be as crucial as the result itself. Effective XAI methods can highlight decision regions in medical images, provide feature importance scores for tabular data, and clarify relationships in multimodal datasets. In this way, XAI not only increases confidence but also helps improve performance, and ensures that AI systems are aligned with clinical needs and standards. In terms of understanding the results of deep learning models, a significant obstacle lies in providing clear explanations for their predictions, especially in crucial areas such as the healthcare field. Several XAI techniques have been developed to tackle this issue, encompassing both *post hoc* and *self-explanatory* methods [20]. Post hoc methods focus on providing explanations for predictions generated by pre-trained black-box models. Among these, model-agnostic approaches have gained significant popularity, as they can be utilized with any black-box model regardless of its internal structure or workings. Several surveys [26, 34] have summarized the usage of XAI techniques in healthcare, providing a comprehensive review of current XAI techniques applied to various types of medical data (e.g., images, text, tabular data, and multimodal) and their applications.

LIME [47] and SHAP [35] are among the most popular XAI techniques. They estimate feature importance by assigning weights, using regression in the case of LIME and a game-theoretic approach for SHAP. In the healthcare field, LIME is widely used to explain prediction results in different scenarios, including the early detection of Parkinson disease [36], prediction of depression symptoms [53], and supporting decisions on lymph node metastasis classification [42]. SHAP is also widely used to support clinical activities such as cancer classification [40], risk of mortality prediction [39], prediction of adverse surgical events [18], and detecting heart anomalies from phonocardiogram (PCG) signals [22]. Similarly, MAPLE (Model-Agnostic Supervised Local Explanations) [43] combines local linear models and ensemble learning methods, such as random forests or gradient-boosted trees, to deliver both accurate predictions and meaningful insights into feature importance. Integrated gradients [51] is a feature attribution approach also used as an XAI method to explain image and language processing [38]. This method evaluates the importance of features by averaging the gradient of the model output, interpolated along a straight-line trajectory in the input data space.

Other XAI techniques have been developed to enhance the interpretability of deep learning models in various application scenarios, including healthcare. GradCAM (Gradient-weighted Class Activation Mapping) [48] is a technique generating visual explanations for convolutional neural network (CNN) models. It produces heatmaps that highlight the regions in medical images (e.g., MRI, X-rays), which can help radiologists in verifying diagnoses and focus areas [37]. Additionally, it is also used to locate abnormalities in electrocardiogram (ECG) or electromyogram (EMG) signals [55]. Layer-wise Relevance Propagation (LRP) [8] is another technique designed to decompose the prediction of a neural network by propagating the output back through the layers to the input features. It assigns relevance scores to each input feature, indicating their contribution to the final prediction. This method has been effectively applied in healthcare for tasks such as image classification [15] and gene expression analysis [19]. Fuzzy classifiers [45] in a different approach to XAI that leverages fuzzy logic theory to provide interpretable rules and reasoning. Such classifiers use fuzzy sets to handle uncertainty and vagueness in data, translating complex model decisions into human-readable rules. In healthcare, fuzzy classifiers can be used in diagnosing diseases or recommending treatments by generating a set of conditional statements (if-then rules) that clinicians can easily understand [17]. Case-based reasoning (CBR) [1] is a XAI technique that explains model predictions by comparing new cases with previously solved cases. In healthcare, CBR can be particularly useful as it mimics human reasoning by drawing analogies between a patient's current situation and past cases stored in a case library. As an example, CBR has been used to identify some factors, including age, hypertension, and urinary infection, which are most effective at predicting renal disease [54].

In contrast, self-explanatory techniques are explicitly designed to generate explanations in tandem with their predictions. However, these approaches often struggle with flexibility and seamless integration into other deep learning frameworks [14, 30]. For example, Bao et al. [10] proposed an explainable AI approach for detecting depressive symptoms in social media using transformer-based models. The authors evaluated single-step and two-step classification-explanation methods, integrating clinical symptom markers and fine-tuned LLMs to enhance interpretability.

However, the main challenge for existing approaches is to find a fair trade-off between accuracy and interpretability of the results [23], with most focusing exclusively on either performance or interpretability. BERT-XDD (BERT-based eXplainable Depression Detection) [13] presents an innovative approach to detecting depression, combining robust classification performance with enhanced interpretability. It leverages BERTweet alongside a bidirectional LSTM equipped with masked attention, providing localized explanations alongside predictions. Additionally, these explanations are further refined into human-readable summaries using ChatGPT, a crucial step for ensuring transparent and comprehensible model decisions in clinical settings where interpretability is essential for fostering trust and usability.

3 A Case Study

In this section, we describe the application of the novel methodology proposed in [13], namely, *BERT-XDD*. This approach provides an accurate and interpretable framework for detecting symptoms of depression in social media users by analyzing the content they have published. As depicted in Fig. 1, BERT-XDD relies on a modular pipeline composed of three main steps:

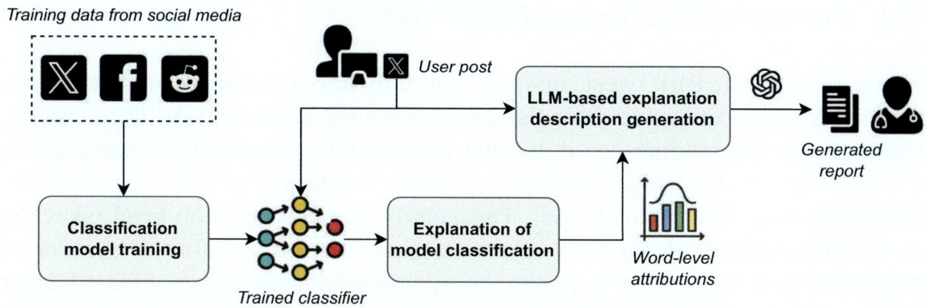

Fig. 1 Overview of the BERT-XDD methodology

- *Classification model training*: the training of a BERT-like classifier for the depression detection task from social media posts.
- *Explanation of model classification*: the application of an XAI technique to determine an explanation at the word level for the model classification (i.e., word attributions).
- *LLM-based explanation description generation*: the use of an autoregressive LLM agent, like OpenAI's ChatGPT or Google Gemini, for the generation of a human-readable report that provides a comprehensive description of the model output based on the user post and the computed explanation.

Thanks to its modularity, this methodology allows full customization, integrating well with different BERT-based classification models and XAI techniques, including self-explanatory and post hoc approaches. Moreover, the choice of the LLM can be tuned according to the available resources and application requirements. In the following sections, we provide a more in-depth description of the main steps of BERT-XDD, describing how it was instantiated in [13], and presenting an application to a Twitter-related case study.

3.1 Self-Explainable Depression Classification

BERT-XDD integrates a novel self-explainable model for depression detection to simultaneously produce classification outcomes and accompanying explanations. Specifically, the approach integrates the BERTweet transformer with a bidirectional LSTM layer enhanced by attention. The training process consists of two distinct steps: first, the *preliminary fine-tuning* of the BERTweet model, followed by the training of the complete *BERT-XDD* model.

3.1.1 Preliminary Fine-Tuning of BERTweet

During this step, the BERTweet classifier is initially fine-tuned on a dedicated corpus of social media posts curated for the depression classification task. The classifier comprises the transformer-based encoder along with a classification head, which processes the resulting logits through a softmax function to produce a probability distribution over the output classes. Particularly, the classification head takes the latent representation of the CLS token computed by the transformer encoder of BERTweet and feeds it to a pooler layer, comprising a fully connected layer followed by a tanh activation. Finally, the pooler output is processed by the output layer, which computes the output vector of logits, normalized through a softmax activation.

The model is trained for 8 epochs with a batch size of 16, using a cross-entropy loss function and a maximum sequence length of 200. Furthermore, among the various neural network optimizers, Rectified Adam with a learning rate of $3 \cdot 10^{-5}$ was chosen to fine-tune the pre-trained weights of BERTweet for the downstream depression detection task [2].

3.1.2 Training of the Complete BERT-XDD Model

In this step, the previously fine-tuned BERTweet model serves as the backbone for building BERT-XDD, a model explicitly designed to generate interpretable outputs using masked attention. Specifically, the BERTweet encoder is retained, while the original classification layer is replaced with a bidirectional LSTM equipped with an attention mechanism. The LSTM computes a weight for each hidden state via a masked attention mechanism, implemented through a parameterized feed-forward neural network, following the approach introduced by Bahdanau et al. [9]. This generates a dynamic score vector, which captures the relative importance of each element in the sequence and serves as unnormalized attention weights for the final classification. Moreover, the attention mechanism leveraged by BERT-XDD employs an attention mask to prevent the model from focusing on irrelevant words for explanation purposes, like stopwords, punctuation, or special tokens like the CLS or PAD. Finally, the BERT-XDD model outputs the predicted class together with an explanation $\mathcal{E}(x)$, represented as a list of pairs $(w_i : \alpha_i)$, where each word w_i is assigned a corresponding attention weight α_i. Such weights indicate the degree of importance the model attributed to each word when making the classification.

The training of the BERT-XDD model involves a two-phase approach. During the first phase, the BERTweet encoder is kept frozen, while optimization is performed solely on the parameters of Bi-LSTM and the masked attention matrices. This optimization process is carried out over six epochs using the ADAM optimizer with a default learning rate of 10^{-3}. In the subsequent phase, the BERTweet encoder is unfrozen, and the complete model undergoes end-to-end fine-tuning for two epochs, following the same configuration used during the initial preliminary fine-tuning stage.

3.2 *Enhancing Model Interpretability Using Large Language Models*

As outlined in earlier sections, one of the main advantages of BERT-XDD is the use of LLMs to translate model explanations into a human-readable format, enabling a thorough understanding of the model decisions. This is particularly useful in clinical settings, where interpretability and transparency are essential for fostering trust and usability of deep learning models.

As described in [13], ChatGPT can be effectively leveraged to transform XAI-based explanations, which consist of a list of word attributions, into a comprehensive and user-friendly report that can be more easily processed by clinical experts. Specifically, the following prompt is used to guide ChatGPT in generating a concise yet meaningful commentary on the classification, based on the input post t, the predicted class that represents the depression level l, and the explanation $E(t)$.

Input Text(\$*t*): {input text coming from a social media post t}
Depression level assigned by classification (\$*l*): {predicted depression class \$*l*}
Explanation (\$e): {list of word-score pairs $(w_i : \alpha_i)$ in $E(t)$}
Role: Act as an expert report writer specializing in social media analysis.
Task: The input will consist of a text (\$t), the predicted depression class \$l, which can be "SEVERELY_DEPRESSED," "MODERATELY_DEPRESSED," or "NOT_DEPRESSED"; an explanation (\$e) as a list of (word: score) pairs sorted in descending order by their relevance on the classification model.

Generate a commentary of 100 words or fewer, quoting the most relevant words from \$(e). Avoid bullet points and additional information beyond what is in \$(e). Do not include any deductions, external context, or opinions. Refer to the following JSON example for guidance:

```
{
    $t: {text t'},
    $l: {class l'},
    $e: {(word : score) in E(t')},
    $c: {example of commentary c'}
}
```

This customized prompt is composed of three main parts:

1. A *task section* that receives as input the text of a post t, the predicted depression level class l, the explanation $E(t)$ (produced by the model as a list of (word: score) pairs, and a set of instructions guiding ChatGPT to create a concise commentary analyzing the class assignment based on the given explanation.

2. A set of *additional instructions* that impose constraints on ChatGPT, limiting the structure and overall length of the generated explanation while preventing personal remarks or unsupported inferences, which is a crucial aspect to preserve transparency in *ChatGPT-augmented* explanations.
3. An *output example* in JSON format, showing ChatGPT how the desired output should be generated, following a one-shot in-context learning approach [16]. Specifically, the prompt includes a sample post t', the predicted depression class l', the explanation $E(t')$ generated by BERT-XDD, and the corresponding example commentary c'.

3.3 Real-World Application to Depression-Related Twitter Posts

In this section, we show some examples of ChatGPT-augmented explanations generated for a Twitter-related case study, encompassing a set of 10,251 posts labeled according to 3 different depression levels, namely, `SEVERELY_DEPRESSED`, `MODERATELY_DEPRESSED`, and `NOT_DEPRESSED`. Analyzed data belong to a dataset made available in [44], which is a preprocessed version of the original one used during the *Shared Task on Detecting Signs of Depression from Social Media Text* competition at LT-EDI-ACL2022 [27].

As an initial example, consider a post that has been correctly classified as `SEVERELY_DEPRESSED`:

> *"Increasing my dose of antidepressants does not help. I was diagnosed with depression from 5 years ago, and ever since, I have been put on meds per the instructions from my shrink. At the beginning, I was only taking one pill of Zoloft a day, but after a few months, I didn't feel any improvements and was still as suicidal as I used to be. I thought the meds didn't work, so I stopped using them for a while. Then things started going into a downward spiral from there. I stopped seeing shrinks and refused to meet any therapist because, deep down inside of me, I have always had this sense of distrust towards anyone beyond my closest circle. I have grown tired of telling them my stories over and over again."*

Beyond predicting the class, the BERT-XDD model also produces an explanation $\mathcal{E}(x)$, which emphasizes the influence of each word on the classification outcome.

$\mathcal{E}(x)$ = {"distrust": 0.1027, "sense": 0.0579, "inside": 0.0258, "closest": 0.0257, "deep": 0.0231, "grown": 0.0224, "thought": 0.0204, "depression": 0.0193, "suicidal": 0.0186, "circle": 0.0162, "beginning": 0.0154, "antidepressants": 0.0154, "tired": 0.0141, "improvements": 0.0141, "stopped": 0.0138, "work": 0.0137, "dose": 0.0134, "shrink": 0.0128, "pill": 0.0128, "diagnosed": 0.0127 }

Building on the model's output, ChatGPT is then used to produce a concise and insightful commentary on the classification through tailored prompts.

Commentary:
"The model identifies the author of this post as `SEVERELY_DEPRESSED`, focusing on "*distrust*", "*suicidal*", and lack of "*improvements*". The author describes feelings "*inside*" their "*closest*" "*circle*", conveying a profound sense of isolation and exhaustion, having "*grown*" "*tired*" of revisiting painful experiences. Words like "*antidepressants*", "*dose*", and "*shrink*" reflect struggles with treatment, while "*stopped*" and "*work*" highlight frustration with ineffective medication. The emphasis on "*deep*" emotions and being "*diagnosed*" with "*depression*" reinforces ongoing distress."

As can be noticed, the generated commentary provides a concise and focused output, highlighting key indicators that succinctly illustrate the severity of the condition. Furthermore, it closely follows the explanation generated by BERT-XDD, which is essential for maintaining the reliability of the generation process.

As a second example, let us analyze another text, which has been correctly identified as `MODERATELY_DEPRESSED`, along with the explanation provided by BERT-XDD:

"*I've got no aspiration, no interest in anything, no fun why do I feel like it takes so much effort to do anything in life. A little background about me: I am a college student. I've been living a decent life with not much trouble in life. Recently I figured out that i might be depressed. i have so much trouble making friends ever since a few years ago. When I meet someone for the first time I try to look cheerful but it gets very tiring and I realized that I avoid gatherings because I find it pointless and tiring.*"

$\mathcal{E}(x)$ = { "depressed": 0.0380, "got": 0.0330, "trouble": 0.0329, "aspiration": 0.0328, "recently": 0.0319, "life": 0.0318, "fun": 0.0302, "background": 0.0290, "gatherings": 0.0283, "decent": 0.0217, "friends": 0.0187, "student": 0.0171, "effort": 0.0170, "living": 0.0155, "feel": 0.0155, "like": 0.0151, "interest": 0.0147, "takes": 0.0143, "college": 0.0136, "figured": 0.0136 }

The analysis provided by ChatGPT is presented below.

Commentary:
"The model identifies the author of this post as `MODERATELY_DEPRESSED`, focusing on "*depressed*", "*aspiration*", and "*trouble*". The author reflects on their "*life*" and "*background*" as a "*college*" "*student*", describing "*effort*" required to engage socially and the absence of "*fun*" or "*interest*". They mention avoiding "*gatherings*" due to "*tiring*" experiences, which contributes to "*trouble*" making "*friends*". The emphasis on "*recently*" and having "*figured*" out their condition highlights emerging self-awareness of being "*depressed*"."

To conclude, let's examine a post labeled as `NOT_DEPRESSED` along with its corresponding analysis.

"*What are you doing when you wanna cry, but do not have a reason? i dunno guys, its kinda weird, but sometimes i have those days when i just wanna cry my eyes out, but i can't find a reason for it, cause i have a good life. It is weird.*"

$\mathcal{E}(x)$ = { "weird": 0.1530, "cry": 0.1284, "life": 0.1034, "cause": 0.1011, "good": 0.0788, "kinda": 0.0559, "guys": 0.0488, "days": 0.0396, "wanna": 0.0374, "reason": 0.0334, "find": 0.0270, "eyes": 0.0183, "dunno": 0.0174 }

Below is the analysis provided by ChatGPT based on the given input.

Commentary:
"The model identifies the author of this post as `NOT_DEPRESSED`, highlighting words such as "*weird*" and "*cry*". The author expresses occasional feelings of wanting to "*cry*" without a clear "*reason*", despite describing their "*good*" "*life*". The use of casual terms like "*guys*", "*kinda*", and "*dunno*" suggests a reflective, conversational tone rather than distress. The focus on "*cause*" and "*reason*" indicates curiosity about fleeting emotions rather than persistent negative feelings, aligning with the model's classification of the post as `NOT_DEPRESSED`."

In all reported cases, the AI-driven augmentation process generated a comprehensive and reliable report that faithfully represents the input explanation in a human-readable format, ensuring trustworthiness. Such commentaries may be useful for clinicians, allowing them to quickly and accurately grasp the insights provided by the explanations. The human-readable format enhances accessibility and facilitates informed decision-making in clinical settings, ultimately improving patient care and treatment strategies.

4 Conclusions

In recent years, research and development activities used machine learning and deep learning techniques to develop AI models of diseases and identify cares for patients. Although some of those approaches are demonstrating accuracy in diagnosis, they provide results without explaining the rationale behind those results. Their use in medicine raises the importance of explaining how these algorithms manage and interpret input data to take informed decisions.

In fact, the lack of transparency poses significant challenges, particularly in the healthcare domain, where decisions can have significant implications for the well-being of patients and treatment paths. This chapter provided an overview of explainable AI techniques for healthcare applications that enable clinicians to better understand and contextualize AI results, and to improve patient care. We also discussed a case study addressing the critical issue of disease detection using social media data, showing how the integration of LLMs with XAI techniques allows to enhance model interpretability, facilitating efficient communication between an AI system and physicians and clinicians.

References

1. Aamodt A, Plaza, E. Case-based reasoning: Foundational issues, methodological variations, and system approaches. AI Commun. 1994;7(1):39–59.
2. Abdulkadirov R, Lyakhov P, Nagornov, N. Survey of optimization algorithms in modern neural networks. Mathematics. 2023;11(11):2466.
3. Abdulsalam A, Alhothali A. Suicidal ideation detection on social media: A review of machine learning methods. Soc Netw Anal Min. 2024;14(1):1–16.
4. Adadi A, Berrada M. Peeking inside the black-box: A survey on explainable artificial intelligence (XAI). IEEE Access. 2019;6:52138–60.
5. Adarsh V, Kumar PA, Lavanya V, Gangadharan G. Fair and explainable depression detection in social media. Inf Process Manag. 2023;60(1):103168.
6. Aishwarya T, Ravi Kumar V. Machine learning and deep learning approaches to analyze and detect covid-19: A review. SN Comput Sci. 2021;2(3):226.
7. Aleem S, Huda Nu, Amin R, Khalid S, Alshamrani SS, Alshehri A. Machine learning algorithms for depression: Diagnosis, insights, and research directions. Electronics. 2022;11(7):1111.
8. Bach S, Binder A, Montavon G, Klauschen F, Müller KR, Samek W. On pixel-wise explanations for non-linear classifier decisions by layer-wise relevance propagation. PloS One. 2015;10(7):e0130140.
9. Bahdanau D, Cho K, Bengio Y. Neural machine translation by jointly learning to align and translate. arXiv preprint arXiv:1409.0473. 2014.
10. Bao E, Pérez A, Parapar J. Explainable depression symptom detection in social media. Health Inf Sci Syst. 2024;12(1):47.
11. Belcastro L, Branda F, Cantini R, Marozzo F, Talia D, Trunfio P. Analyzing voter behavior on social media during the 2020 US presidential election campaign. Social Network Analysis and Mining. 2022;12:83.
12. Belcastro L, Cantini R, Marozzo F. Knowledge discovery from large amounts of social media data. Appl Sci. (Switzerland). 2022;12(3). https://doi.org/10.3390/app12031209.
13. Belcastro L, Cantini R, Marozzo F, Talia D, Trunfio P. Detecting mental disorder on social media: a ChatGPT-augmented explainable approach. Online Social Networks and Media. 2025;48:100321.
14. Bhargava P, Ng V. Commonsense knowledge reasoning and generation with pre-trained language models: A survey. In Proceedings of the AAAI Conference on Artificial Intelligence. Online Conference, 2022;36:12317–12325.
15. Binder A, Bockmayr M, Hägele M, Wienert S, Heim D, Hellweg K, Ishii M, Stenzinger A, Hocke A, Denkert C, et al. Morphological and molecular breast cancer profiling through explainable machine learning. Nat Mach Intell. 2021;3(4):355–66.
16. Brown T, et al. Language models are few-shot learners. Adv Neural Inf Proces Syst. 2020;33:1877–1901.
17. Cao J, Zhou T, Zhi S, Lam S, Ren G, Zhang Y, Wang Y, Dong Y, Cai J. Fuzzy inference system with interpretable fuzzy rules: Advancing explainable artificial intelligence for disease diagnosis–a comprehensive review. Inf Sci. 2024;662:120212.
18. Chen H, Lundberg SM, Erion G, Kim JH, Lee SI. Forecasting adverse surgical events using self-supervised transfer learning for physiological signals. NPJ Digital Med. 2021;4(1):167.
19. Chereda H, Bleckmann A, Menck K, Perera-Bel J, Stegmaier P, Auer F, Kramer F, Leha A, Beißbarth T. Explaining decisions of graph convolutional neural networks: Patient-specific molecular subnetworks responsible for metastasis prediction in breast cancer. Genome Med. 2021;13:1–16.
20. Das A, Rad P. Opportunities and challenges in explainable artificial intelligence (XAI): A survey. arXiv preprint arXiv:2006.11371. 2020.

21. De Fauw J, Ledsam JR, Romera-Paredes B, Nikolov S, Tomasev N, Blackwell S, Askham H, Glorot X, O'Donoghue B, Visentin D, et al. Clinically applicable deep learning for diagnosis and referral in retinal disease. Nat Med. 2018;24(9):1342–50.
22. Dissanayake T, Fernando T, Denman S, Sridharan S, Ghaemmaghami H, Fookes C. A robust interpretable deep learning classifier for heart anomaly detection without segmentation. IEEE J Biomed Health Inform. 2020;25(6):2162–71.
23. Dziugaite GK, Ben-David S, Roy DM. Enforcing interpretability and its statistical impacts: Trade-offs between accuracy and interpretability. arXiv preprint arXiv:2010.13764. 2020.
24. Govindasamy, KA, Palanichamy, N. Depression detection using machine learning techniques on twitter data. In 2021 5th International Conference on Intelligent Computing and Control Systems (ICICCS) (pp. 960–966). IEEE. 2021.
25. Hasib KM, Islam MR, Sakib S, Akbar MA, Razzak I, Alam MS. Depression detection from social networks data based on machine learning and deep learning techniques: An interrogative survey. IEEE Trans Comput Social Syst. 2023;10(4):1568–86.
26. Hossain MI, Zamzmi G, Mouton PR, Salekin MS, Sun Y, Goldgof D. Explainable AI for medical data: Current methods, limitations, and future directions. ACM Comput Surv; 2023. https://doi.org/10.1145/3637487
27. Kayalvizhi S, Thenmozhi D. Data set creation and empirical analysis for detecting signs of depression from social media postings. In: Computational intelligence in data science. Cham: Springer International Publishing; 2022. pp. 136–51.
28. Ker J, Bai Y, Lee HY, Rao J, Wang L. Automated brain histology classification using machine learning. J Clin Neurosci. 2019;66:239–45.
29. Kerasiotis M, Ilias L, Askounis D. Depression detection in social media posts using transformer-based models and auxiliary features. Soc Netw Anal Min. 2024;14(1):196.
30. Kumar P, Raman B. A bert based dual-channel explainable text emotion recognition system. Neural Netw. 2022;150:392–407.
31. Liu M, Hu L, Tang Y, Wang C, He Y, Zeng C, Lin K, He Z, Huo, W. A deep learning method for breast cancer classification in the pathology images. IEEE J Biomed Health Inform. 2022;26(10):5025–32.
32. Liu Y, Jain A, Eng C, Way DH, Lee K, Bui P, Kanada K, de Oliveira Marinho G, Gallegos J, Gabriele S, et al. A deep learning system for differential diagnosis of skin diseases. Nat Med. 2020;26(6):900–8.
33. Liu-Zarzuela J, Munoz I, Truong N, Zahra A, Mallya M, Grayson K. Postpartum depression and facebook: A cross-sectional study of content quality and reliability. J Affect Disord Rep. 2024;16:100745.
34. Loh HW, Ooi CP, Seoni S, Barua PD, Molinari F, Acharya UR. Application of explainable artificial intelligence for healthcare: A systematic review of the last decade (2011–2022). Comput Methods Prog Biomed. 2022;226:107161. https://doi.org/10.1016/j.cmpb.2022.107161. https://www.sciencedirect.com/science/article/pii/S0169260722005429
35. Lundberg SM, Lee SI. A unified approach to interpreting model predictions. Adv Neural Inf Proces Syst. 2017;30:4765–4774.
36. Magesh PR, Myloth RD, Tom RJ. An explainable machine learning model for early detection of parkinson's disease using lime on datscan imagery. Comput Biol Med. 2020;126:104041.
37. Mahesh TR, Vinoth Kumar V, Guluwadi, S. Enhancing brain tumor detection in MRI images through explainable AI using grad-cam with resnet 50. BMC Med Imaging. 2024;24(1):107.
38. Makino MEA. The impact of integration step on integrated gradients. In: Proceedings of the 18th conference of the european chapter of the association for computational linguistics: Student research workshop, St. Julian's; 2024. pp. 279–89.
39. Na Pattalung T, Ingviya T, Chaichulee S. Feature explanations in recurrent neural networks for predicting risk of mortality in intensive care patients. J Perinat Med. 2021;11(9):934.
40. Nahiduzzaman M, Abdulrazak LF, Ayari MA, Khandakar A, Islam SR. A novel framework for lung cancer classification using lightweight convolutional neural networks and ridge extreme learning machine model with shapley additive explanations (shap). Expert Syst Appl. 2024;248:123392.

41. O'Dea B, Boonstra TW, Larsen ME, Nguyen T, Venkatesh S, Christensen H. The relationship between linguistic expression in blog content and symptoms of depression, anxiety, and suicidal thoughts: A longitudinal study. Plos one. 2021;16(5):e0251787.
42. Palatnik de Sousa I, Maria Bernardes Rebuzzi Vellasco M, Costa da Silva, E. Local interpretable model-agnostic explanations for classification of lymph node metastases. Sensors. 2019;19(13):2969.
43. Plumb G, Molitor D, Talwalkar AS. Model agnostic supervised local explanations. Adv Neural Inf Proces Syst. 2018;31:2520–2529.
44. Poświata R, Perełkiewicz M. Detecting signs of depression from social media text using RoBERTa pre-trained language models. In: 2nd workshop on language technology for equality, diversity and inclusion, Dublin; 2022. pp. 276–82.
45. Prokopowicz P, Czerniak J, Mikolajewski D, Apiecionek L, Slezak D. Theory and applications of ordered fuzzy numbers. Springer Nature Cham, Switzerland; 2017.
46. Qasrawi R, Polo SPV, Al-Halawa DA, Hallaq S, Abdeen Z, et al. Assessment and prediction of depression and anxiety risk factors in schoolchildren: Machine learning techniques performance analysis. JMIR Formative Res. 2022;6(8):e32736.
47. Ribeiro MT, Singh S, Guestrin C. "Why should i trust you?" Explaining the predictions of any classifier. In: 22nd ACM SIGKDD, San Francisco; 2016. pp. 1135–44.
48. Selvaraju RR, Cogswell M, Das A, Vedantam R, Parikh D, Batra D. Grad-cam: Visual explanations from deep networks via gradient-based localization. In: Proceedings of the IEEE international conference on computer vision, Venice; 2017. pp. 618–26.
49. Senn S, Tlachac M, Flores R, Rundensteiner E. Ensembles of bert for depression classification. In: 2022 44th annual international conference of the IEEE engineering in Medicine & Biology Society (EMBC), Glasgow. IEEE; 2022. pp. 4691–4.
50. Sumathi M, Poorna B. Prediction of mental health problems among children using machine learning techniques. Int J Adv Comput Sci Appl. 2016;7(1):552–557.
51. Sundararajan M, Taly A, Yan Q. Axiomatic attribution for deep networks. In: International conference on machine learning, Sydney; 2017. PMLR, pp. 3319–28.
52. Talia D, Trunfio P, Marozzo F, Belcastro L, Cantini R, Orsino A. Programming big data applications: Scalable tools and frameworks for your needs, 2024. ISBN: 978-1-80061-504-5
53. Uddin MZ, Dysthe KK, Følstad A, Brandtzaeg PB. Deep learning for prediction of depressive symptoms in a large textual dataset. Neural Comput Appl. 2022;34(1):721–44.
54. Vásquez-Morales GR, Martinez-Monterrubio SM, Moreno-Ger P, Recio-Garcia JA. Explainable prediction of chronic renal disease in the colombian population using neural networks and case-based reasoning. IEEE Access. 2019;7:152900–10.
55. Wickstrøm K, Mikalsen KØ, Kampffmeyer M, Revhaug A, Jenssen R. Uncertainty-aware deep ensembles for reliable and explainable predictions of clinical time series. IEEE J Biomed Health Inform. 2020;25(7):2435–44.
56. Wongkoblap A, Vadillo MA, Curcin V. Social media big data analysis for mental health research. In: Stein DJ, Fineberg NA, Chamberlain SR, editors. Mental Health in a Digital World. Global Mental Health in Practice. Academic Press; 2022. p. 109–143.

Part II
Techniques and Methodologies

Batch-Integrated Gradients: A Library for Explaining Temporal Health Data

Jamie Duell, Hsuan Fu, and Xiuyi Fan

Contents

Abstract Deep Learning methods are often utilised for medical predictions, but they suffer from a lack of interpretability, thus the demand for transparent and interpretable models has become imperative. However, while methods for explaining model decisions have been extensively explored, temporal explanations remain largely underrepresented. To address this gap, we propose the Batch-Integrated Gradients (Batch-IG) library, building upon the foundation of the Integrated Gradients method. Batch-IG aims to provide temporal explanations by attributing the model's predictions of input features over time. By integrating gradients along the temporal dimension, Batch-IG offers insights into how changes in input features contribute to model predictions across time batches. Our method extends the applicability of integrated gradients to temporal domains, thereby enhancing the interpretability of deep learning models operating on temporal data. This chapter presents a simple

J. Duell (✉) · X. Fan
Lee Kong Chian School of Medicine, Nanyang Technological University, Singapore, Singapore
e-mail: jamie.duell@ntu.edu.sg; xyfan@ntu.edu.sg

H. Fu
Department of Finance, Insurance and Real Estate, Université Laval, Quebec, QC, Canada
e-mail: hsuan.fu@fsa.ulaval.ca

R. Ortale et al. (eds.), *Explainable Machine Intelligence in Healthcare*,
https://doi.org/10.1007/978-3-031-91379-2_5

library for applying Batch-Integrated Gradients for Neural Networks developed in PyTorch.

Keywords Explainable AI · Deep learning · Integrated gradients

1 Introduction

Deep learning is a common method that is utilized for medical predictions [1]. Unfortunately, deep learning architectures often lack transparency in their predictions, and thus Explainable Artificial Intelligence (XAI) is a field that gained popularity with landmark papers introducing the Local Interpretable Model-Agnostic Explanations (LIME) method by Ribeiro et al. [2] and the SHapley Additive exPlanations (SHAP) method by Lundberg and Lee [3]. These approaches are model-agnostic and rely on approximating the decision boundary given by prediction models. For deep learning approaches, XAI methods such as integrated gradients (IG) [4] utilize the continuous and differentiable form of neural networks to produce explanations. These methods fall under the feature attribution umbrella of XAI techniques that aim to answer the question:

> *For a prediction generated by a machine learning method, which features were deemed significant?*

Feature attribution techniques in medical data analysis yield valuable insights into the relative importance of different features, which can be instrumental in addressing critical questions in clinical settings [12]. These techniques have been instrumental for various prediction problems, including cancer mortality prediction [5], cancer metastasis prediction [6], and drug sensitivity prediction [7], among others [8].

The occurrence of temporal data can often be seen in healthcare [9], but many existing XAI methods do not account for the temporal nature of the data [10]. As existing feature attribution algorithms in XAI [11] cannot directly answer this question, as they treat each record as an independent instance and do not consider temporal changes.

To this end, we propose the Batch-Integrated Gradients (Batch-IG) library to facilitate open-source research and provide a simple implementation of the Batch-IG method for neural networks that are developed using the PyTorch[1] framework, extending on our previous work in [13–15].

The rest of the chapter is organized as follows: Section 2 provides details on the IG architecture and how it is extended to Batch-IG. Section 3 provides a simple comparison to DeepSHAP. Section 4 provides implementation details that contain code examples for the implementation of Batch-IG.

[1] https://pytorch.org/

2 From Integrated Gradients to Batch-Integrated Gradients

2.1 Integrated Gradients

Given an instance to explain $\mathbf{x} = \langle x^1, \ldots, x^m \rangle \in X$, where $X \in \mathbb{R}^{n \times m}$ is a dataset, the IG [4] formulation, presents a feature attribution method for accumulating and averaging gradients on a straight line path between a baseline $\mathbf{x}'$ and an instance to explain $\mathbf{x}$. The IG approach considers an all-zero vector $\mathbf{x}'$ baseline, such that $\mathbf{x}' = \langle 0^1, \ldots, 0^J \rangle$.

Formally, let $F : \mathbb{R}^m \rightarrow [0, 1]$ represent a deep network, a smooth function $\psi = \langle \psi^1, \ldots, \psi^m \rangle : [0, 1] \rightarrow \mathbb{R}^m$, which takes an input $\tau \in [0, 1]$ and maps to a m-dimensional point along a smooth path that traverses from the baseline instance $\mathbf{x}'$ to an instance $\mathbf{x}$. Thus, attribution is calculated by integrating over a path $\psi(\tau)$ for $\tau \in [0, 1]$. The path-integrated gradients formulation is defined as

$$\text{Path-IG}_j^{\psi}(\mathbf{x}) = \int_{\tau=0}^{1} \frac{\partial F(\psi(\tau))}{\partial \psi^j(\tau)} \frac{\partial \psi^j(\tau)}{\partial \tau} d\tau,$$

where IG is a unique case of Path-IG that adheres to a straight line path $\mathbf{x}' + \tau(\mathbf{x} - \mathbf{x}')$ where

$$\text{IG}_j(\mathbf{x}) = (x^j - x'^{,j}) \times \int_{\tau=0}^{1} \frac{\partial F(\mathbf{x}' + \tau(\mathbf{x} - \mathbf{x}'))}{\partial x^j} d\tau.$$

2.2 Batch-Integrated Gradients

To construct Batch-Integrated Gradients, we first consider the Interval Integrated Gradients (IIG) method [14] that considers temporal data between any two time points; we present this idea in Fig. 1. Thus, given a temporal dataset $X^t = \langle \mathbf{x}, b \rangle$, where $\mathbf{x}$ is an instance and b is the time batch index $\chi_b \subseteq X^t$. Then, $\mathbf{x}_t \in \chi_b$ is a time point for $t \in [1 : T]$, where T is the number of time points in χ_b. The IIG formulation considers two instances $\mathbf{x}_t$ and $\mathbf{x}_{t+1}$ of a batch χ_b and describes a linear interpolation between two time points; this can be described over a single j^{th} dimension as

$$\text{IIG}_j(\mathbf{x}_{t+1}, \mathbf{x}_t) = (x_{t+1}^j - x_t^j) \times \int_{\tau=0}^{1} \frac{\partial F(\mathbf{x}_t + \tau(\mathbf{x}_{t+1} - \mathbf{x}_t))}{\partial x_t^j} d\tau.$$

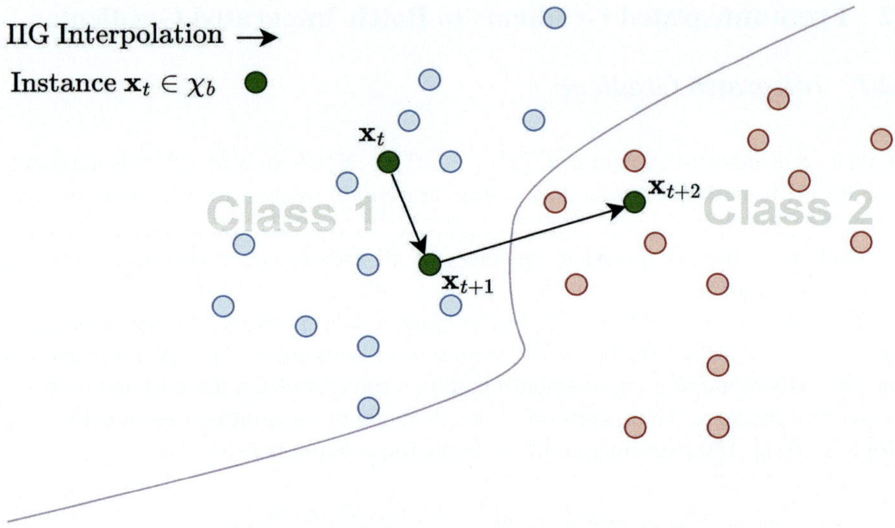

Fig. 1 Simple illustration of the Batch-IG method, accumulating IIG explanations over linear interpolations for each instance within in a time batch χ_b

The Batch-IG form is then a simple extension to consider all attributions over a time batch χ_b, and is thus defined over the jth feature dimension for a straight line path between temporal points as

$$\begin{aligned}\text{Batch-IG}_j(\chi_b) &= \sum_{t=1}^{T-1} \text{IIG}_j(\mathbf{x}_{t+1}, \mathbf{x}_t) \\ &= \sum_{t=1}^{T-1} (x_{t+1}^j - x_t^j) \times \int_{\tau=0}^{1} \frac{\partial F(\mathbf{x}_t + \tau(\mathbf{x}_{t+1} - \mathbf{x}_t))}{\partial x_t^j} d\tau.\end{aligned}$$

Since this approach falls under the family of path integral methods, we can rewrite the IIG formulation over all j dimensions, by considering the gradient of F, namely, ∇F, over a path and relax the straight line path definition and consider any path between time points. Thus, we let γ represent a path between $\mathbf{x}_t$ and $\mathbf{x}_{t+1}$, where $[\mathbf{x}_t, \mathbf{x}_{t+1}]$ is the interval that γ traverses. The function ψ maps to a point τ in this interval. We then write the IIG formulation as

$$\int_\gamma \nabla F \cdot d\psi = \int_{\mathbf{x}_t}^{\mathbf{x}_{t+1}} \nabla F(\psi(\tau)) \cdot \psi'(\tau) d\tau.$$

Here, $F(\psi(\tau))$ is our neural network F applied to a function that maps to an interpolation point τ along a path from $\mathbf{x}_t$ to $\mathbf{x}_{t+1}$, where our integral is evaluated with respect to a change in τ; thus, for the straight line interpolation is equivalent to evaluating our function along a path over the path $F(\mathbf{x}_t + \tau(\mathbf{x}_{t+1} - \mathbf{x}_t))$. The $\psi'(\tau)$ term represents the first derivative of our path function with respect to our interpolation along a path between $\mathbf{x}_t$ and $\mathbf{x}_{t+1}$, in other words determining how each dimension of the instance $\mathbf{x}_t$ changes with respect to a change in the interpolation τ. Thus, one is evaluating:

$$\psi'(\tau) = \left\langle \left(\frac{dx_t^1}{d\tau}\right), \ldots, \left(\frac{dx_t^m}{d\tau}\right) \right\rangle,$$

this formulation implies, from the additive property of integrals, that over all dimensions j, Batch-IG computes:

$$\begin{aligned}\int_\gamma \nabla F \cdot d\psi &= \int_{\mathbf{x}_t}^{\mathbf{x}_T} \nabla F(\psi(\tau)) \cdot \psi'(\tau) d\tau \\ &= \int_{\mathbf{x}_t}^{\mathbf{x}_{t+1}} \nabla F(\psi(\tau)) \cdot \psi'(\tau) d\tau \; + \ldots + \int_{\mathbf{x}_{T-1}}^{\mathbf{x}_T} \nabla F(\psi(\tau)) \cdot \psi'(\tau) d\tau.\end{aligned}$$

Therefore, this equivalence the Batch-IG method can effectively capture the difference in prediction probabilities between time points over a time batch, since

$$\int_{\mathbf{x}_t}^{\mathbf{x}_T} \nabla F(\psi(\tau)) \cdot \psi'(\tau) d\tau = F(\mathbf{x}_T) - F(\mathbf{x}_t). \tag{1}$$

Similarly, IIG captures the prediction probabilities between any two time points $\mathbf{x}_t$ and $\mathbf{x}_{t+1}$, since

$$\int_{\mathbf{x}_t}^{\mathbf{x}_{t+1}} \nabla F(\psi(\tau)) \cdot \psi'(\tau) d\tau = F(\mathbf{x}_{t+1}) - F(\mathbf{x}_t). \tag{2}$$

Equations 1 and 2 illustrate how both IIG and Batch-IG capture the attribution values associated with the difference in prediction between time points. Batch-IG and IIG leverage two essential properties: *time completeness* and *time sensitivity*. Informally, time completeness ensures that the feature attribution values across two time points capture the difference in predictions between those points. Meanwhile, time sensitivity guarantees that features remaining constant over time receive no attribution. Formal details of this are presented in [14].

2.3 Computing Batch-Integrated Gradients

For the computation of Batch-IG, we first define the Riemann approximation for the IIG method; this is defined as

$$\mathrm{IIG}_j^{\mathcal{R}}(\mathbf{x}_t, \mathbf{x}_{t+1}) = (x_{t+1}^j - x_t^j) \times \frac{1}{K} \sum_{k=1}^{K} \frac{\partial F(\mathbf{x}_t + \frac{k}{K} \times (\mathbf{x}_{t+1} - \mathbf{x}_t))}{\partial x^j},$$

where K is the number of steps for the Riemann approximation. The approximation satisfies time completeness as we show by representing straight line between time points as

$$\theta_K^j = \frac{1}{K} \sum_{k=1}^{K} \frac{\partial F(\mathbf{x}_t + \frac{k}{K} \times (\mathbf{x}_{t+1} - \mathbf{x}_t))}{\partial x^j}.$$

As K approach infinity, then:

$$\Big(F(\mathbf{x}_{t+1}) - F(\mathbf{x}_t)\Big) - \Big(\sum_{j=1}^{m} \theta_K^j (x_{t+1}^j - x_t^j)\Big) = 0,$$

implies time completeness. Time sensitivity is satisfied if $x_{t+1}^j = x_t^j$, since the IIG formulation computes:

$$\theta_K^j \times 0 = 0,$$

over the jth feature dimension. To extrapolate to the Batch-IG formulation, we sum over the number of time steps to cover a batch χ_b; this is defined as

$$\begin{aligned}\text{Batch-IG}_j^{\mathcal{R}}(\chi_b) &= \sum_{t=1}^{T-1} \mathrm{IIG}_j^{\mathcal{R}}(\mathbf{x}_t, \mathbf{x}_{t+1}) \\ &= \sum_{t=1}^{T-1} (x_{t+1}^j - x_t^j) \times \frac{1}{K} \sum_{k=1}^{K} \frac{\partial F(\mathbf{x}_t + \frac{k}{K} \times (\mathbf{x}_{t+1} - \mathbf{x}_t))}{\partial x^j}.\end{aligned}$$

3 Explanation Similarities

This chapter uses artificial data from the Simulacrum, a synthetic dataset developed by Health Data Insight CiC and derived from anonymous cancer data provided by the National Disease Registration Service, NHS England. We used subsets of

Table 1 Comparison of explanations returned by DeepSHAP and Batch-IG$^{\mathcal{R}}$

Dataset	Average correlation	Correlation std.	Correlation var.
Breast Cancer	0.52	0.22	0.05
Lung Cancer	0.71	0.30	0.09
Rectal Cancer	0.44	0.24	0.06
Lymphoma Cancer	0.67	0.27	0.07
Skin Cancer	0.46	0.27	0.07

medical data derived from the Simulacrum dataset, focusing on various types of cancer such as lung cancer, breast cancer, rectal cancer, lymphoma, and skin cancer. Each subset was identified according to the corresponding ICD-10 codes for these cancers.[2]

We compare the explanations returned by Batch-IG$^{\mathcal{R}}$ and DeepSHAP, by evaluating the average Pearson correlation coefficient r of the explanation vectors returned over the first 100 instances in 5 datasets, where the DeepSHAP approximation background set uses the whole training dataset and Batch-IG$^{\mathcal{R}}$ uses $K = 5000$ steps for the Riemann approximation. Due to Batch-IG computation, Batch-IG utilizes the difference term computed by $\mathbf{x}_{t+1} - \mathbf{x}_t$, where any feature of the same value between sequential time points within a batch of time points is assigned zero-value attribution between time points.

To extend, we compare the similarity of explanations produced for the ANN model by both Batch-IG and DeepSHAP. Since the DeepSHAP method only produces feature attribution explanations for individual instances without considering the temporal aspect within our EHR data, we manually take the difference between two instances at each adjacent time interval and consider that as the impact of changes. We observe that there is a moderate to high average correlation between explanations returned by Batch-IG$^{\mathcal{R}}$ and DeepSHAP across the majority of datasets with a relatively large standard deviation (see Table 1).

4 Implementation Details

4.1 Package Details

In Table 2, we present the metadata for the Batch-IG library introduced in this chapter.

[2] https://simulacrum.healthdatainsight.org.uk/

Table 2 Code metadata

Code metadata description	Details
Current code version	v1.0.0
Legal Code License	MIT License
Software code languages, tools, and services used	Python
Dependencies	Dependencies: PyTorch, NumPy, SciPy, matplotlib.
Library link	https://pypi.org/project/batch-integrated-gradients/
GitHub link	https://github.com/jamie-duell/batch_integrated_gradients

4.2 Functions

The Batch-IG library requires a pip installation, which can be executed using the following:

```
pip install batch_integrated_gradients
```

after installing Batch-IG, we initialise Batch Integrated Gradients, with the following, where we pass the pretrained PyTorch neural network:

```
    batch_integrated_gradients = BatchIntegratedGradients(model)
```

We then select an instance index to explain, the input tensor that contains the instance, the number of time steps we wish to explain, and the number of steps in the Riemann approximation (100 in the example) of the Batch-IG method and extract the calculated values from Batch-IG.

```
batch_ig_values =
     batch_integrated_gradients.BatchIG_values(initial_index,
     input_tensor, time_steps, n_steps=100)
```

This returns the batch-integrated gradient values, the prediction probabilities associated with each interpolation, and all values of the gradient along each path. This then allows us to plot two forms of explanation visualizations:

- The Batch-IG summary plot.
- The Batch-IG gradient plot.

The Batch-IG gradient plot provides a simple plot for a selection of features, determined by the feature indices. For example, consider the feature indices:

$$[0, 1, 2, 3, 4, 5, 6, 7, 8, 9, 10, 11, 12],$$

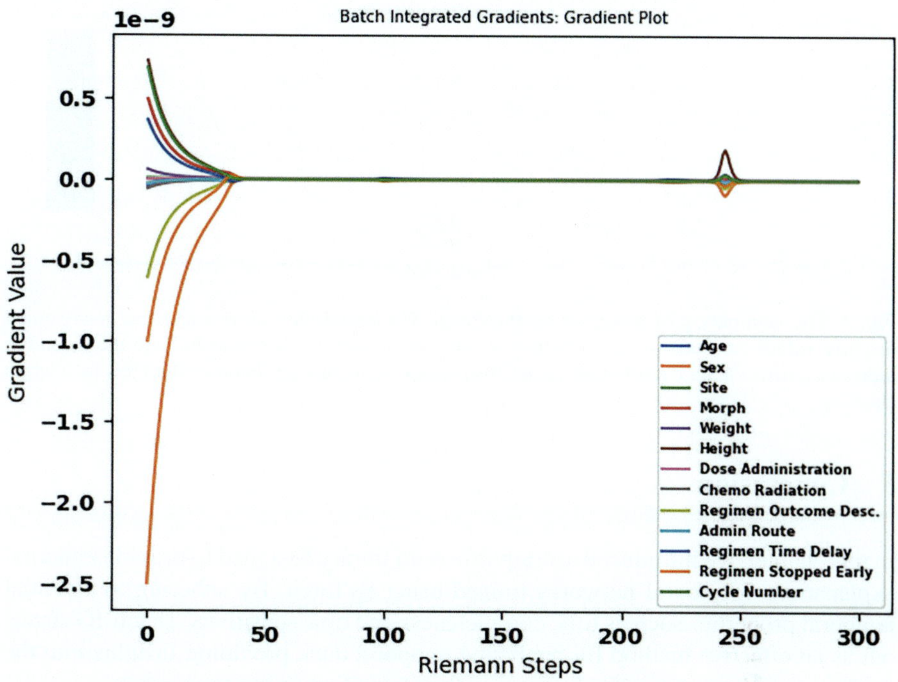

Fig. 2 The gradient plot produced over IIG explanations that accumulate to the Batch-IG explanation. These gradients are highlighted with their associated gradient value and the corresponding Riemann step on the linear interpolation. Each color represents a patient feature

the gradient plot associated with these features is implemented with:

```
selected_feature_indices = [0,1,2,3,4,5,6,7,8,9,10,11,12]
batch_integrated_gradients.GradientPlot(batch_ig_values[2],
    feature_names, selected_feature_indices)
```

The explanation is presented in Fig. 2; here we observe how each features gradients are mapped along time intervals over $K \cdot T$ Riemann steps. The summary plot function provides a bar plot of the calculated Batch-IG values, and is implemented with:

```
selected_feature_indices = [0,1,2,3,4,5,6,7,8,9,10,11,12]
batch_integrated_gradients.SummaryPlot(batch_ig_values[0], feature_names,
    selected_feature_indices)
```

Using this, we then generate the explanation illustrated in Fig. 3. Here we observe that the Batch-IG method captures the dynamic and static features over the time batch, where attribution is only assigned to the features: dose administration, admin route, and cycle number.

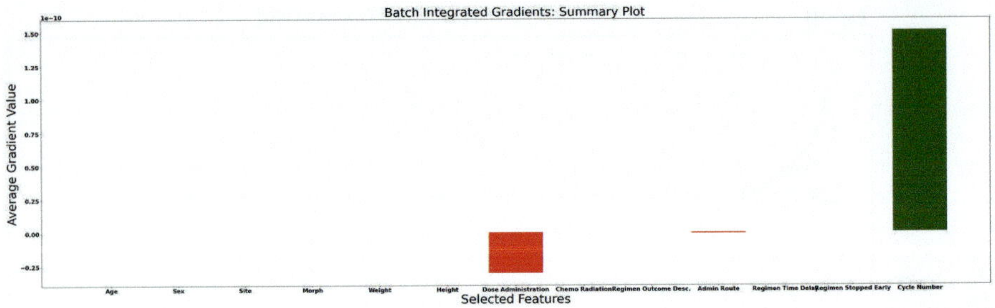

Fig. 3 The summary plot produced by the Batch-IG method, this summarizes the positive and negative values attributed for a collection of time points within a time batch. Here the green bar indicates positive feature attribution values (resp. negative feature attribution value) toward a target class

5 Conclusion

In this chapter, we introduced a straightforward library designed to provide temporal explanations for neural networks trained using PyTorch. By adhering to essential temporal properties such as time completeness and time sensitivity, Batch-IG stands out as an effective method for analyzing temporal data, providing insights into the attribution of importance for features as they transition over a time batch.

This chapter includes a straightforward empirical evaluation of time sensitivity applied to a controlled dataset with known attribution. We emphasize that Batch-IG accurately assigns zero-value attribution to features that remain constant over time. Additionally, we conduct a basic Pearson correlation analysis, revealing a medium to high correlation across various synthetic medical datasets, indicating similarities in the assigned feature attribution between DeepSHAP and Batch-IG.

We provide clear examples of explanations generated using Batch-IG to illustrate the explanation process. This enables easy observation of the gradients linked with Batch-IG explanations and visualization of the feature attribution produced by Batch-IG.

References

1. Kapcia M, et al. ExMed: An AI tool for experimenting explainable AI techniques on medical data analytics. In: IEEE 33rd international conference on tools with artificial intelligence, Washington, DC. 2021.
2. Ribeiro M, et al. “Why Should I Trust You?”: Explaining the predictions of any classifier. In: Proceedings of the 22nd ACM SIGKDD international conference on knowledge discovery and data mining, San Francisco. 2016.
3. Lundberg S, et al. A unified approach to interpreting model predictions, advances in NeurIPS 30. In: Annual conference on NeurIPS, Long Beach, CA. 2017.

4. Sundararajan M, et al. Axiomatic attribution for deep networks. In: Proceedings of the 34th international conference on machine learning, Sydney. 2017.
5. Duell J, et al. A comparison of explanations given by explainable artificial intelligence methods on analysing electronic health records. In: IEEE EMBS international conference on biomedical and health informatics, Athens. 2021.
6. Yagin B, et al. Cancer metastasis prediction and genomic biomarker identification through machine learning and eXplainable Artificial Intelligence in breast cancer research. Diagnostics (Basel). 2023 Oct 26;13(21):3314. https://doi.org/10.3390/diagnostics13213314. PMID: 37958210; PMCID: PMC10650093
7. Gillani S, et al. Explainable AI in drug sensitivity prediction on cancer cell lines. In: International conference on emerging trends in smart technologies, Karachi. 2022.
8. Shahab S, et al. Application of explainable artificial intelligence in medical health: A systematic review of interpretability methods. Inf Med Unlock. 2023;40:101286
9. Batal I, et al. A temporal pattern mining approach for classifying electronic health record data. ACM Trans Intell Syst Technol. 2013;4(4):1–36. https://doi.org/10.1145/2508037.2508044
10. Simic I, et al. XAI methods for neural time series classification: A brief review, arXiv. 2021.
11. Loh HW, et al. Application of explainable artificial intelligence for healthcare: A systematic review of the last decade (2011–2022). Comput Methods Programs Biomed. 2022;226:1–21. 107161. https://doi.org/10.1016/j.cmpb.2022.107161
12. Amann J, et al. Explainability for artificial intelligence in healthcare: A multidisciplinary perspective. BMC Med Inform Decis Mak. 2020;20:310. https://doi.org/10.1186/s12911-020-01332-6
13. Duell J, Fan X, Fu H, Seisenberger M. Batch integrated gradients: explanations for temporal electronic health records. In: Juarez JM, Marcos M, Stiglic G, Tucker A, editors. Artificial intelligence in medicine. AIME 2023. Lecture notes in computer science. vol 13897. Cham: Springer. https://doi.org/10.1007/978-3-031-34344-5_15
14. Duell, J. et al. A formal introduction to batch-integrated gradients for temporal explanations. In: IEEE 35th international conference on tools with artificial intelligence, Atlanta, GA. 2023.
15. Duell J. Explainable artificial intelligence for medical science, Swansea University, 2024.

Decision Tree Models to Select High-Risk Patients for Lung Cancer Screening and Model Interpretability

Teena Rai, Yuan Shen, Jaspreet Kaur, Jun He, Mufti Mahmud, David J. Brown, David R. Baldwin, Emma O'Dowd, and Richard Hubbard

Contents

T. Rai · Y. Shen · J. He (✉) · M. Mahmud · D. J. Brown
Department of Computer Science, Nottingham Trent University, Nottingham, UK
e-mail: teena.rai2022@my.ntu.ac.uk; yuan.shen@ntu.ac.uk; jun.he@ntu.ac.uk; mufti.mahmud@ntu.ac.uk; david.brown@ntu.ac.uk

J. Kaur · D. R. Baldwin · E. O'Dowd · R. Hubbard
Division of Epidemiology and Public Health, University of Nottingham, Nottingham, UK
e-mail: jaspreet.kaur1@nottingham.ac.uk; david.baldwin@nottingham.ac.uk; emma.odowd@nottingham.ac.uk; richard.hubbard@nottingham.ac.uk

R. Ortale et al. (eds.), *Explainable Machine Intelligence in Healthcare*,
https://doi.org/10.1007/978-3-031-91379-2_6

Abstract Lung cancer is the most common cause of cancer deaths in the UK emphasizing the critical need for early diagnosis. Survival rates vary significantly according to the stage of diagnosis. This study aims to develop machine learning models to classify between lung cancer and non-lung cancer cases using data from the Clinical Practice Research Datalink (CPRD) which includes UK primary care records. Both interpretable and post hoc explainable approaches are explored including RuleFit, a rule-based method; decision tree, an inherently interpretable model; and random forest and eXtreme Gradient Boosting, tree-based ensemble models. The model performance is assessed using metrics such as accuracy, Area Under the Receiver Operating Characteristic Curve, sensitivity, and specificity. The models performed similarly across all measures. Additionally, SHapley Additive exPlanations (SHAP) and Local Interpretable Model-agnostic Explanations (LIME) are employed to enhance model interpretability. These insights contribute to better understanding the leading risk factors for lung cancer. Using SHAP, it is found that age and smoking status play a crucial role in lung cancer prediction for all tree-based models. Then, LIME is used to evaluate individual-level explanations and identify any discrepancies in their explanations between different models. Our study combines robust evaluation with prominent interpretability techniques to gain valuable insights into lung cancer prediction.

Keywords Decision tree · Lung cancer · Risk prediction · Global interpretation · Local interpretation

1 Introduction

1.1 Background

Lung cancer is the third most common cancer in the UK [5], and around 48,500 people were diagnosed with lung cancer every year between 2016 and 2018. It is also the most common cause of cancer deaths in the UK. According to [5], the 5-year net survival of people who were diagnosed with stage I lung cancer between 2016 and 2020 was 65% compared to only 5% if they were diagnosed at an advanced stage. Therefore, it is crucial to diagnose people with lung cancer at an early stage to help save lives.

In 2006, UK National Screening Committee (NSC) did not recommend screening for lung cancer due to insufficient evidence supporting the usefulness of screening. However, in 2022 UK NSC recommended targeted screening for lung cancer across the UK [27]. They looked at publications up to June 2021 and found evidence based on randomized control trials (RCTs) that people with lung cancer benefited from screening. For example, their evidence review included results from the NELSON trial [17] where participants between the ages of 50 and 74 were recruited from regions in the Netherlands and Belgium between 2003 and 2005. Participants were randomly subjected to low-dose computed tomography (LDCT) screening in years

1, 3, and 5.5 (screening groups) from 2004 to 2012 and without screening (control group). At 10 years of follow-up, the cumulative incidence of lung cancer was 5.58 cases per 1000 person-years in the screening group and 4.91 cases per 1000 person-years in the control group. Furthermore, cumulative lung cancer mortality was 2.50 deaths per 1000 person-years in the screening group compared to 3.30 deaths in the control group showing that lung cancer mortality was significantly lower between the screening groups compared to the control groups. Therefore, it is essential to identify people at high risk of lung cancer so that they can be referred for screening to ensure timely detection and intervention for those most susceptible to it.

1.2 Objectives of the Study

The main objectives of this chapter are:

1. Develop inherently interpretable machine learning models, including RuleFit and Decision Trees (DTs), as well as two tree-based ensemble models – random forest (RF) and eXtreme Gradient Boosting (XGB). Compare their performance metrics, such as Area Under the Receiver Operating Characteristic Curve (AUROC), accuracy, sensitivity, and specificity.
2. Employ two prominent post hoc model-agnostic approaches such as SHapley Additive exPlanations (SHAP) and Local Interpretable Model-agnostic Explanations (LIME) – to explain predictions made by the ensemble models.
3. Compare the explainability provided by inherently interpretable models with that of model-agnostic approaches.

2 Related Work

There have been particularly two well-known regression-based risk prediction models for lung cancer: the Liverpool Lung Project (LLP) risk model [6] and $PLCO_{m2012}$ [25]. For the LLP risk model, 579 people with lung cancer and 1157 controls were recruited from the Liverpool area between 1998 and 2005 where a questionnaire was used to collect their information on socioeconomic and demographic characteristics, medical history, family history of cancer, history of tobacco consumption, and lifetime occupational history. These risk factors were used to build the logistic regression model that gave an AUROC of 0.70 with sensitivity of 62% and specificity of 70% at 2.5% classification threshold and sensitivity of 34% and specificity of 90% at 6% threshold. For the $PLCO_{m2012}$ model, participants were aged between 55 and 74 years with any smoking status. There were almost equal number of participants in the control (77,456) and intervention (77,445) groups, and the AUROC for smokers in the control group was 0.803 and the intervention group was 0.797 with sensitivity of 83% and specificity of 62.9%.

The LLP risk model and the $PLCO_{m2012}$ model have been well validated in external datasets [23, 26]. There has been growing research to build machine learning models for the prediction of lung cancer risk with increased accuracy and AUROC. In [10], demographic characteristics, smoking information, BMI data, and laboratory data were used to develop XGB that performed better than $PLCO_{m2012}$ with an AUROC of 0.86 and had increased accuracy in identifying lung cancer among ever-smoker up to 12 months before clinical diagnosis (p-value <0.00001). Similarly, primary care datasets from CPRD have been used to develop risk prediction models with several machine learning classifiers for esophagogastric cancer [4], and their performance has been compared with the current UK esophagogastric cancer risk-assessment tool (ogRAT). All predictive models (random forest, linear SVM, logistic regression, naive Bayes, and XGBoost) used in this paper outperformed ogRAT with their accuracy at 89%.

Recent research has increasingly focused on enhancing machine learning interpretability using techniques like SHAP and LIME. For instance, in a study that applied well-validated regression-based lung cancer models (PLCOm2012 [25], BACH [2], and LCRAT [15]) to real patient data from the Polish population [16], age and smoking-related variables emerged as the top predictors of lung cancer risk. While these features were globally important across all models, their impact on individual patients varied, emphasizing the need to understand personalized model predictions. Additionally, rule extraction techniques such as RuleFit [9] have been employed to create interpretable ensemble classifiers in other domains, including finance for credit scoring [1]. These studies have furthered the aims and objectives of this study.

3 Decision Tree Models

Decision tree, RuleFit, random forests, and eXtreme Gradient Boosting are used for the classification task. We use [11, 14] to explain the theory behind them in this section.

3.1 Decision Tree

A decision tree is made of a collection of nodes and edges where the root node holds all of the training data and each decision node is further split into disjoint subsets of the training data on all available features depending on the tests associated with each decision node. This procedure is repeated until all nodes of the tree are leaf nodes or a stopping criterion is reached.

There are different algorithms to grow a decision tree. We use Classification and Regression Tree (CART) to grow a decision tree which adopts binary node splitting and uses the Gini index as its splitting criterion of the internal nodes. The Gini index refers to the probability of misclassification of a certain randomly selected feature. It is defined as

$$\text{gini(S)} = \sum_{i=1}^{c} p_{ik}(1 - p_{ik}) = \sum_{i=1}^{c} p_{ik} - \sum_{i=1}^{c}(p_{ik})^2 = 1 - \sum_{i=1}^{c}(p_{ik})^2,$$

where c represents the number of classes in the target variable and p_{ik} represents the number of training observations in the k-th node that belongs to the class i.

The Gini index of the split is the weighted average of the Gini index across the decision sub-nodes of S. Hence, a lower Gini index value corresponds to lower likelihood of misclassification. So once we identify the split along a feature with the lowest Gini index, we split the root node across that specific feature and similarly split other decision nodes until all nodes of the tree are leaf nodes or a stopping criterion is reached.

Entropy can be used an alternative splitting criterion which is defined as

$$\text{Entropy(S)} = -\sum_{i=1}^{c} p_{ik}(1 - p_{ik})$$

where p_{ik} and c are defined as above. Similar to the Gini index, a small value of entropy indicates that a node contains observations which are primarily from a single class.

3.2 Random Forest

RF uses bagging to build an ensemble of decision tree classifiers, where each tree is trained on a randomly selected bootstrap subset of the training data. Instead of choosing a random subset of features at the tree level, RF selects a random subset of features at each node. This ensures diversity in how the model learns the relationships between features. Hence, for each tree, a random bootstrap sample is drawn from the training set with replacement and at each node, a random subset of features is selected to ensure variability across trees. The node is then split based on a defined criterion (e.g., Gini or entropy as defined above) to form a decision tree from the sample. This process is repeated to generate n decision trees, each producing a prediction, and the final output is determined by aggregating the predictions through majority voting.

3.3 XGBoost

Unlike random forest, which uses bagging, XGB employs boosting to build an ensemble model by sequentially training weak learners, primarily decision trees. The process begins with an initial prediction from the first decision tree, assigning a weight to its output. In subsequent iterations, XGB increases the weight of data points that were misclassified by previous trees, ensuring the model focuses on correcting errors. This weighted data is then passed to the next tree in the sequence. Gradient boosting enhances this approach by applying the gradient descent algorithm to optimize the iterative learning process of weak models. Although boosting is typically sequential, XGB speeds up the process by constructing trees in parallel, significantly improving computational efficiency.

Figure 1 clarifies the difference between bagging and boosting. Furthermore, [11] gives a good introduction to decision tree-based models.

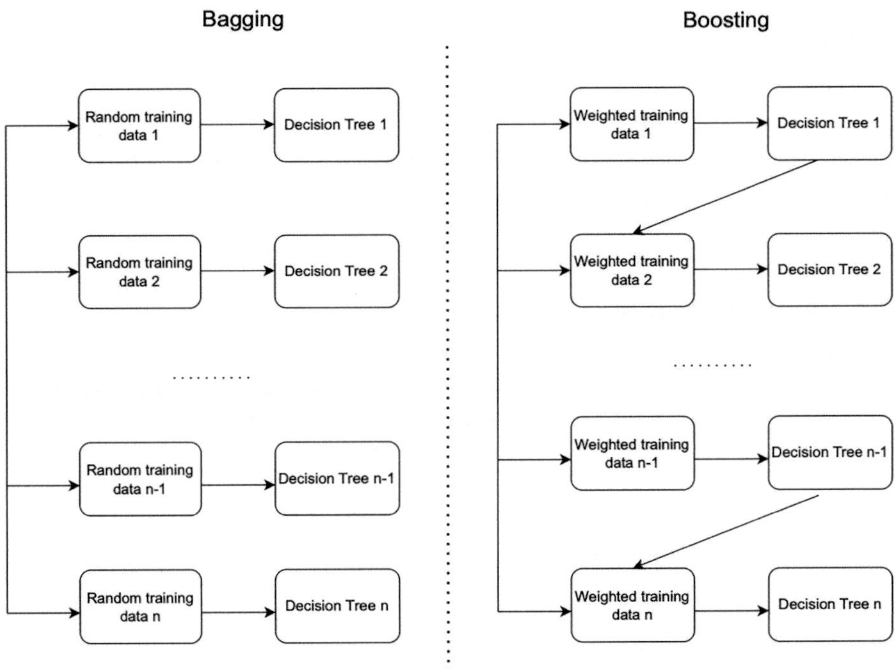

Fig. 1 Difference between bagging and boosting. Models are trained in parallel in bagging whereas models are trained sequentially in boosting

3.4 Decision Rules

In this section, we will introduce an additional interpretable model known as decision rules. We will look into the details of decision rules in this section using [20]. Decision rules consist of simple IF-THEN statements with conditions that can be made to make predictions. A simple example could be IF it is a weekday AND it is 8 a.m., THEN coffee sales are high. Therefore, decision rules can be described as one of the most interpretable models because it mirrors the way people think and make decisions.

Let us look at a hypothetical example of predicting ice cream sales. A decision rule for this prediction task could be if temperature is greater than 20 °C and it is a weekend, then the sale of ice cream is high, i.e., IF "temp >20" AND "day = weekend," THEN "sale = high." We can measure the usefulness of this decision rule in terms of its support and accuracy.

The support of a rule is defined as the percentage of the observations to which the conditions of the decision rule applies to. For our above decision rule for predicting ice cream sales, suppose for 15 out of 100 observations, the temperature was greater than 20 °C and it was a weekend; then, the support of the rule is 15%. The accuracy of a rule is defined as the percentage of observations it correctly classifies when the condition of the rule is applied. For example, out of the 100 observations where "temp >20" AND "day = weekend," THEN "sale = high" applies, 80 have "sale = high," then the accuracy of the rule is 80%.

We will be looking at a particular form of decision rule called RuleFit [9] which generates new features from the original ones in the form of decision rules to capture interaction between the features. It then fits a linear model with the original features and new features as input. Hence, we have an interpretable linear model which integrates feature interactions. Note that in this chapter, our primary focus when using RuleFit is on interpretability rather than evaluating model performance.

A collection of decision rules are generated using decision trees. Gradient boosting as described in Sect. 3 is used to fit an ensemble of decision trees with the original features. Multiple decision rules are constructed from each tree in the ensemble. Let s_j be the set of all possible values for input variable x_j, then $x_j \in s_j$ and $s_{jm} \subset s_j$. We create rules of the following form from all the trees in the ensemble:

$$r_m(x) = \prod_{j \in T_m} I(x_j \in s_{jm}) \tag{1}$$

where m is one of the decision trees in the ensemble, T_m is the set of features used in the m-th tree and I(.) is an indicator function:

$$I(x_j \in s_{jm}) = \begin{cases} 1 \text{ if } x_j \in s_{jm} , \\ 0 \text{ if } x_j \notin s_{jm}. \end{cases}$$

The decision rules as described in Eq. 1 and the original features are used to train a linear model with the following structure:

$$F(x) = \hat{a}_0 + \sum_{k=1}^{K} \hat{a}_k r_k(x) + \sum_{j=1}^{p} \hat{\beta}_j l_j(x_j) \tag{2}$$

where $\hat{a}$ and $\hat{\beta}$ are the coefficients for the decision rules and original features respectively estimated using L1 regularized linear regression model on the training data.

Additionally, when it comes to decision rules, their importance is determined using the following formula:

$$I_k = |\hat{a_k}|.\sqrt{s_k(1 - s_k)} \tag{3}$$

where $\hat{a_k}$ is the associated coefficient of the decision rule as described in Eq. 2 and s_k is the support of the rule, as described earlier.

Hence, decision trees are inherently interpretable models because we can observe the decision process by following the nodes of the tree. We will see this concept in practice in Sect. 6.2. In contrast, interpreting RF and XGB is more challenging. In subsequent sections, we employ both model-specific and model-agnostic approaches to interpret these complex models.

4 Data and Methods

4.1 Data Overview and Preprocessing

The real-world UK primary care CPRD GOLD data [12] was used to develop the machine learning models in this study. CPRD consists of anonymized patient information from over 600 general practitioners (GPs) all over the UK with information about over 10 million patients. The cohort comprised of men and women aged between 50 and 80 years. Each patient was followed from January 1, 2014 until one of the events occurred for the patient – death date, diagnosis of lung cancer, or end of the follow up period, January 1, 2020. The final data comprised of 1,414,134 healthy controls and 10,757 lung cancer cases.

The features used in this study are listed below:

1. Age (`age`) is categorized into six groups: 50–54, 55–59, 60–64, 65–69, 70–74, 75–79.
2. Smoking status (`smoking_status`) was categorized as Current or Ex Unknown, Ex Unknown, Ex Light, Ex Moderate, Ex Heavy, Current Unknown, Current Light, Current Moderate, Current Heavy.

3. Alcohol status (alcohol_status) was categorized as Never, Ex Unknown, Ex Non Heavy, Ex Heavy, Current Unknown, Current Non Heavy, Current Heavy.
4. BMI (bmi) was categorized as Underweight, Normal, Overweight, Obese, and Morbidly Obese.
5. Presence or absence of the following symptoms: dyspnea (dyspnea), hemoptysis (haemoptysis), and sputum (sputum).
6. Weightloss (weightloss) is a binary variable indicating if patients reported any weightloss.
7. Family history of cancer (family_history_of_cancer) and family history of lung cancer (family_history_of_lung_cancer) are binary variables indicating if patient had any family history of cancer and family history of lung cancer, respectively.
8. COPD referred as Chronic Obstructive Pulmonary Disease (copd) is a binary variable indicating the presence or absence of COPD.
9. Presence or absence of personal history of individual cancer – head and neck cancer (head_and_neck_cancer), bladder cancer (bladder_cancer), pancreatic cancer (pancreatic_cancer), thyroid cancer (thyroid_cancer), stomach cancer (stomach_cancer), kidney cancer (kidney_cancer), leukemia (luekemia), ovary cancer (ovary_cancer), myeloma (myeloma), melanoma (melanoma).
10. lungcancer is a binary target variable to denote lung cancer cases and non-lung cancer cases.

Given that we are working with primary care data, which is not routinely collected for research purposes, our dataset contains missing values for several features. Specifically, we have missing values for smoking_status, alcohol_status, and bmi. To handle these missing values, we recode them as "missing." Additionally, we apply ordinal encoding to the features age, smoking_status, alcohol_status, and bmi, maintaining the same order as described earlier, with the value "missing" assigned the lowest order.

4.2 Methodology

The dataset is split into five folds using stratified shuffle split, ensuring that each fold maintains the same class distribution. For each fold, 10% of the data is reserved for testing, while the remaining folds are used for training. Specifically, we have 1,263,452 non-lung cancer cases and 9268 lung cancer cases for training, and 140,338 non-lung cancer cases and 1076 cases for testing in each fold. This results in a highly imbalanced dataset, where lung cancer cases are significantly outnumbered by non-lung cancer cases. The lung cancer instances constitute only 0.0076% of the data. A similar methodology has also been implemented as in our previous work [21, 22] to address this class imbalance using a modified undersampling technique based on [18]. We ensure an equal number of non-lung cancer cases, and lung cancer

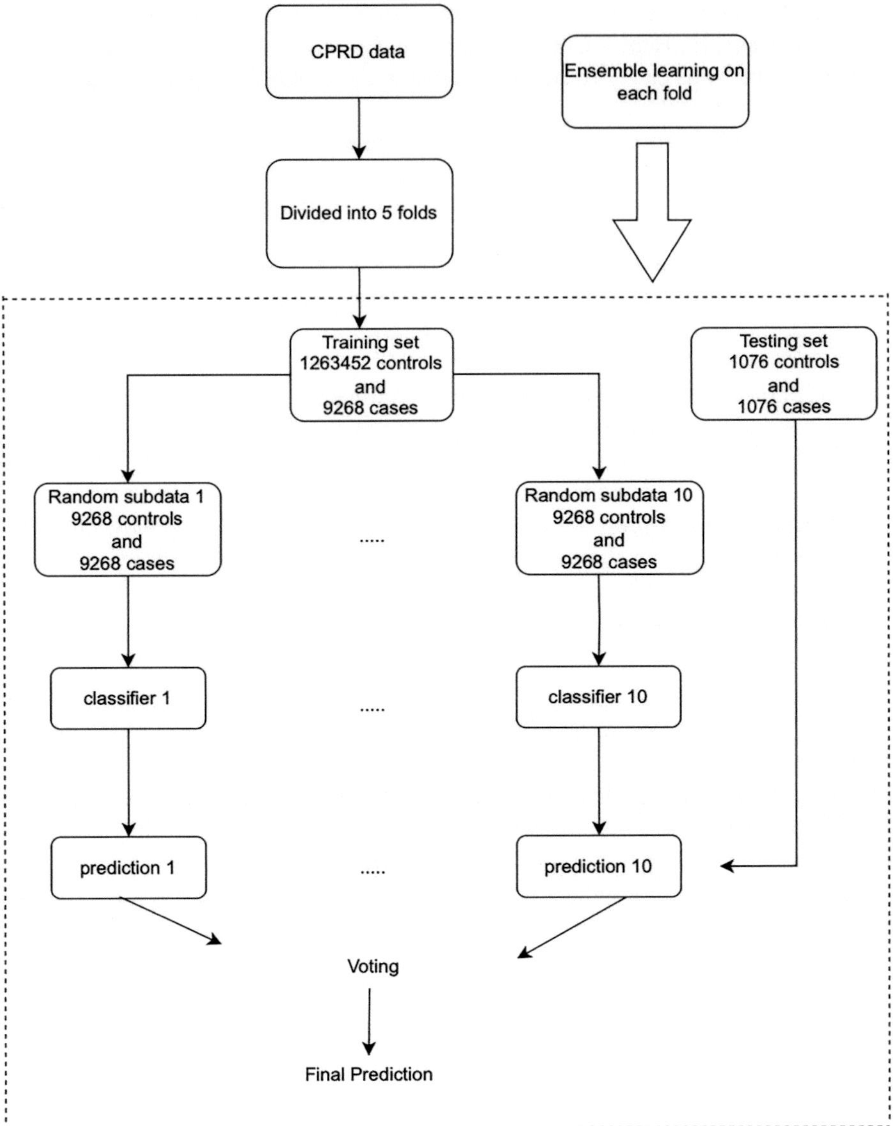

Fig. 2 Undersampling in an ensemble setting

cases are sampled from the training folds, as depicted in Fig. 2. Subsequently, each classifier is trained using this balanced dataset, and predictions are generated using the test set, which also maintains a balanced distribution. This process is repeated ten times, with lung cancer cases and a distinct sample of non-lung cancer cases randomly drawn from the training dataset for each iteration. The final predictions for the testing data are determined through majority voting based on the ten predicted labels from each classifier. Figure 2 visually illustrates this procedure, and the average performance of the models across all folds is reported in this study.

4.3 Hyperparameter Tuning

In the field of machine learning, hyperparameters refer to external configuration parameters that are manually set before training a model to optimize its performance. Unlike internal parameters such as coefficients in a logistic regression model that are learned during the training process, hyperparameters are predefined. Before training the models in this chapter, we prioritize tuning specific hyperparameters to optimize overall model performance.

For DT, we tune the following hyperparameters:

1. maximum depth of the tree, `max_depth` - `range(2, 10)`,
2. splitting criterion, `criterion` - `{'gini', 'entropy'}`.

For RF, the following hyperparameters are tuned:

1. `max_depth` - `range(2, 10)`,
2. `criterion` - `{'gini', 'entropy'}`,
3. The number of trees (estimators) in the forest, `n_estimators` - `{100, 200, 300, 500}`,
4. Minimum number of samples required to split an internal node, `min_samples_split` - `{300, 400, 600}`.

For XGB, the following hyperparameters are tuned:

1. `max_depth` - `range(2, 10)`,
2. `n_estimators` - {100, 200, 400, 500},
3. learning rate which controls the weight of each tree added to the model, `learning_rate` - `{0.01, 0.1, 0.3}`.

We conducted a grid search, exhaustively exploring all specified parameter combinations, using fivefold cross-validation to identify the optimal hyperparameters for our models. The hyperparameters that yielded the highest accuracy were subsequently employed for model training. Specifically, for DT, the maximum accuracy was achieved with a maximum depth of 8 and the entropy criterion. RF achieved its highest accuracy with a maximum depth of 9, the entropy criterion, 300 estimators, and a minimum sample split of 400. XGB attained maximum accuracy with a maximum depth of 4, a learning rate of 0.1, and 200 estimators.

5 Interpretability

5.1 Feature Importance Methods

In our analysis of lung cancer prediction, we employ two post hoc feature importance methods, SHAP and LIME for interpreting ensemble-based models. SHAP provides insights into both global and individual-level feature importance. On the other hand, LIME focuses on explaining individual predictions. While we provide a concise explanation of the theory behind SHAP and LIME below, we recommend referring to [20] for a more comprehensive understanding of these concepts.

5.1.1 SHAP

SHAP [19] can be used to interpret any model in terms of their global and local feature importances. The underlying theory of SHAP draws from Shapley values in coalitional game theory, which are used to determine fair payouts in scenarios where each participant contributes differently. In the context of prediction tasks, each feature within an observation can be likened to a "player" in a game, and its predicted value represents the "payout." The Shapley value is computed by taking the difference between the predicted value of coalition with and without the features which gives the marginal contribution of each feature. These values are then averaged over all possible combination of features to get a Shapley value for each feature.

5.1.2 LIME

LIME [24] uses local surrogate models to approximate the individual predictions of any black box model. The process starts by selecting a specific observation of interest. The original data is then perturbed to generate a new dataset, along with the corresponding predictions. LIME fits an interpretable model (e.g., linear regression) to this perturbed data, where the model's weights are influenced by the proximity of the altered samples to the observation being explained, providing a localized understanding of the prediction.

6 Results

6.1 Model Evaluation

The models are compared in terms of their accuracy, AUROC, sensitivity, and specificity. All tree-based models exhibited comparable performance across various evaluation metrics, as summarized in Table 1. Among them, XGB outperformed the others in terms of accuracy, AUROC, and specificity.

We firstly present the interpretation given by DT in the form of a tree structure with nodes and branches. For ensemble models, interpretability is achieved using SHAP and LIME. These methods shed light on the predictive behavior of complex models from different angles. Additionally, we utilize RuleFit, a decision rule-based approach, to identify the most critical rules that influenced the model's predictions. Note that to simplify interpretation and reduce computation time, we select one of the models from our ensemble setting as depicted in Fig. 2 for applying interpretability techniques.

6.2 *Interpretation of Decision Trees and Decision Rules*

DTs are interpretable because we can trace the decision path and gain insight into how the model reached a specific decision. We will now explore the decision tree that was generated during the training process.

Interpretation of Fig. 3: The decision tree begins with the root node containing all the training data. It then splits into two sub-nodes based on the feature `smoking_status` chosen because it has the lowest entropy among all features. These sub-nodes hold disjoint subsets of the training data. The process continues by calculating feature entropies and selecting the lowest one to split the sub-nodes. This repetition occurs until all nodes become leaf nodes or a predefined stopping criterion is met. By setting a maximum depth of 8 for this model, the tree stops expanding once it reaches that threshold.

The tree in Fig. 3 is plotted using `scikit-learn` module in Python. However, the `dtreeviz` Python module offers enhanced visualization capabilities for decision trees as depicted in Fig. 4.

In Fig. 4, the distribution of lung cancer and non-lung cancer cases becomes more evident. Since age was encoded using ordinal encoding (with increasing age having a higher order), we observe from the stacked bar chart that as both age and smoking status increase, the incidence of lung cancer cases also rises.

We will now utilize RuleFit to identify the top rules employed by the model in its predictions. Our focus lies on enhancing interpretability, rather than evaluating model performance.

The top five rules based on importance as described in Eq. 3 are generated using RuleFit as follows:

Table 1 Performance evaluation

Classifiers	Accuracy	AUROC	Sensitivity	Specificity
DT	67.59	0.75	68.22	66.97
RF	67.91	0.75	68.97	66.82
XGB	68.96	0.76	67.62	70.30

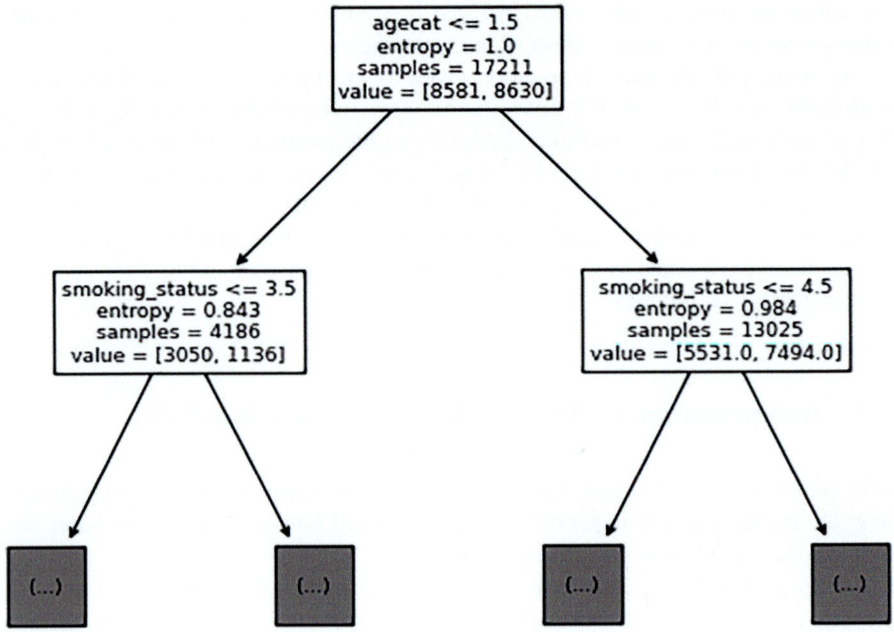

Fig. 3 Decision tree created during the training process. The maximum depth of the tree has been intentionally limited to a maximum depth of 1 for simplicity

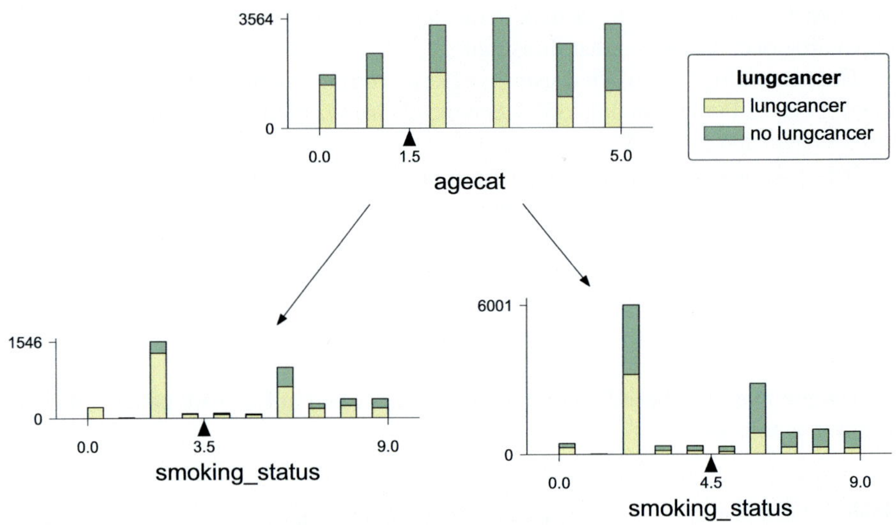

Fig. 4 Visualization of DT in Fig. 3 using `dtreeviz` module with maximum depth set to 1 for simplicity

Rule 1: `smoking_status` > 1.5 and `age` > 0.5
Rule 2: `smoking _status` <= 2.5 and `COPD` <= 0.5
Rule 3: `breast_cancer` <= 0.5 and `smoking_status` <= 7.5 and `COPD` <= 0.5
Rule 4: `weightloss` <= 0.5 and `sputum` <= 0.5 and `alcohol_status` <= 6.5 and `alcohol_status` > 5.5
Rule 5: `haemoptysis` <= 0.5 and `weightloss` <= 0.5 and `sputum` <= 0.5 and `kidney_cancer` <= 0.5 and `bladder_cancer` <= 0.5 and `smoking_status` <= 8.5

Interpretation of Rule 1: The combination of `smoking_status` ∈ {"Ex Unknown," "Ex Light," "Ex Moderate," "Ex Heavy," "Current Unknown," "Current Light," "Current Moderate," "Current Heavy"} and `age` ∈ {"55–59," "60–64," "65–69," "70–74," "75–79"} plays the most important rule in distinguishing between lung cancer and non-lung cancer cases. This rule has a high support (occurring frequently in the dataset) of 86.96%. Additionally, its accuracy – measuring how well it predicts the correct class for instances satisfying its condition – on the testing set is 66.6%. Given that this accuracy is comparable to previous models, it suggests that this rule plays a crucial role in the classification of lung cancer cases.

Similarly, we can analyze the remaining rules in this manner. Their accuracies fall within the range of 66.12–67.86%. These rules collectively contribute to the overall classification performance. However, it is important to note that as additional conditions are incorporated into the decision rules, although the accuracy of the rule improves, the support of the rule diminishes. Consequently, the decision rules become more restrictive and challenging to interpret. For example, consider Rule 5: the support is 77.67% and its accuracy stands at 67.86%.

Hence, RuleFit focuses on global interpretability, aiming to provide an overall understanding of the entire model through decision rules. In contrast to SHAP and LIME, RuleFit generates rules that are easy for humans to understand that describe how the input features impact the model's predictions.

6.3 Global Interpretation of Ensemble Models Using SHAP

We will now explore the use of SHAP and LIME to interpret the ensemble models. It is important to note that both SHAP and LIME can be applied to any model, including inherently interpretable models like decision trees. However, in this study, we specifically focus on comparing the native interpretability of decision trees with the explanations provided by SHAP and LIME. Additionally, we will begin by using SHAP to assess the overall feature importance for a global model interpretation. Subsequently, we will examine individual predictions using LIME to check their alignment. While SHAP can also explain individual predictions, our primary goal is to introduce a variety of interpretability methods applicable to our prediction task.

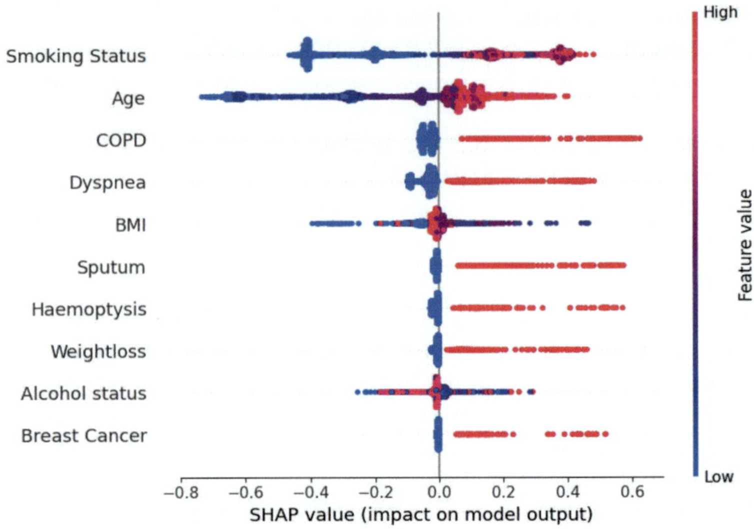

Fig. 5 SHAP values across all test data points for RF

We calculate SHAP values for the test dataset to visualize how they vary across all features and multiple data points, providing a global interpretation of the model. By analyzing SHAP values across all test data points, we gain insight into feature importance, interactions, and overall model behavior. In Figs. 5 and 6, the top ten features in predicting lung cancer risk are depicted. The x-axis represents the SHAP values, while the y-axis shows the features. The color indicates the features' value, ranging from low to high. Since our dataset contains only categorical variables and we've implemented ordinal encoding, higher SHAP values correspond to the order mentioned in Sect. 4.1. In the plot, features are ranked based on importance, defined as the average of absolute SHAP values per feature across the data. Each dot represents the SHAP value of the respective feature for that specific data point.

In Figs. 5 and 6, we see that the features `smoking_status` and `age` stand out as the most influential factors regarding the classification of lung cancer versus non-lung cancer cases. As `age` increases, the corresponding SHAP value also increases. Similarly, as `smoking_status` increases, the SHAP value also rises. Therefore, higher categories of `age` and `smoking_status` positively influence the prediction of lung cancer. When dealing with binary variables such as COPD, symptoms and personal and family history of cancer (as outlined in Sect. 4.1 of our preprocessing steps), presence of a feature is coded as 1 and absence of a feature is coded as 0 to ensure consistency. Hence, we observe that presence of `copd` and symptoms such as `dyspnea`, `haemoptysis`, and `sputum` play a positive role in the prediction of lung cancer. This observation aligns with existing literature [7, 8]. The distribution of BMI values shows clusters with both high- and low-order feature values, particularly centered around the plot. This observation suggests that BMI may not be a highly relevant feature for prediction in our context. The personal history of breast cancer is

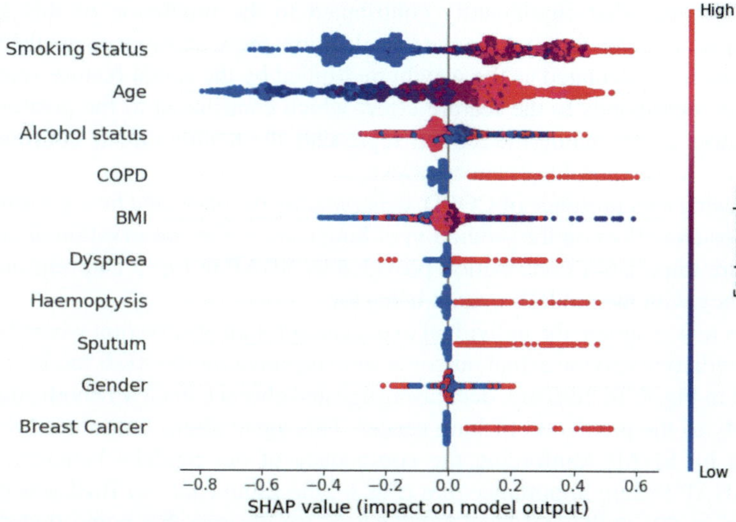

Fig. 6 SHAP values across all test data points for XGB

the only cancer which appears in the top ten most important features. Interestingly, women with a history of breast cancer seem to play a positive role in predicting lung cancer. This observation aligns with existing literature [3, 13] although warrants further investigation.

Therefore, SHAP values offer a clear understanding of how individual features contribute to model predictions. The global feature importance derived from SHAP provides insights into the model's decision-making process. Moreover, we saw that they help interpret black box models (like ensembles) by revealing feature effects. While DT models inherently provide a tree structure for interpretation, SHAP values go beyond. SHAP values reveal both positive and negative contributions made by features. DTs are more interpretable in the sense that they display decision-making processes similar to human reasoning. Depending on the problem, this humanlike interpretability can be advantageous. In summary, SHAP values provide a clear lens for understanding model intricacies, while DTs offer a more intuitive decision-making representation.

6.4 Local Interpretation of Ensemble Models Using LIME

Global explanations as outlined in Sect. 6.3 offer insights into the overall behavior of a model. On the other hand, individual-level explanations allow us to understand predictions for specific instances or observations.

We firstly examine the individual explanation for an observation where both the model prediction and the actual outcome were positive for the RF model. The top five features that significantly contributed to the prediction of this specific observation are given in Fig. 7. In the visualization, the x-axis represents the feature effect, which is calculated as the weight multiplied by the actual feature value. The green bar corresponds to the feature effect which contributed to the positive class (lung cancer cases), while the red bar represents the feature effects contributed to the negative class (non-lung cancer cases).

Increasing age, presence of COPD, experiencing dyspnea, and heavy smoking all have a positive effect on the prediction of lung cancer. This observation aligns with the feature importance contribution provided by SHAP in Fig. 5 and reinforces the consistency with the model's overall behavior.

Let us now examine the individual explanation for an observation where both the model prediction and the actual outcome were negative for the XGB model which is depicted in Fig. 8. In this case, decreasing age and absence of COPD both contribute negatively to the prediction of lung cancer. This again aligns with the explanation provided by SHAP, reinforcing the consistency of our model's behavior. In the global SHAP feature importance plot (Fig. 6), the significance of BMI was unclear. However, in this individual-level explanation, we observe that being underweight has positively contributed to the prediction. This emphasizes the importance of understanding individual-level factors in our model's predictions.

Let us now explore an observation where the RF model predicted a positive outcome, but the actual result turned out to be negative. This scenario is depicted in Fig. 9. In such cases, understanding why the model made an incorrect prediction can provide valuable insights for model improvement and decision-making. In this case, the presence of sputum and increasing age has particularly influenced the model's positive prediction which is consistent to the SHAP explanation depicted in Fig. 5.

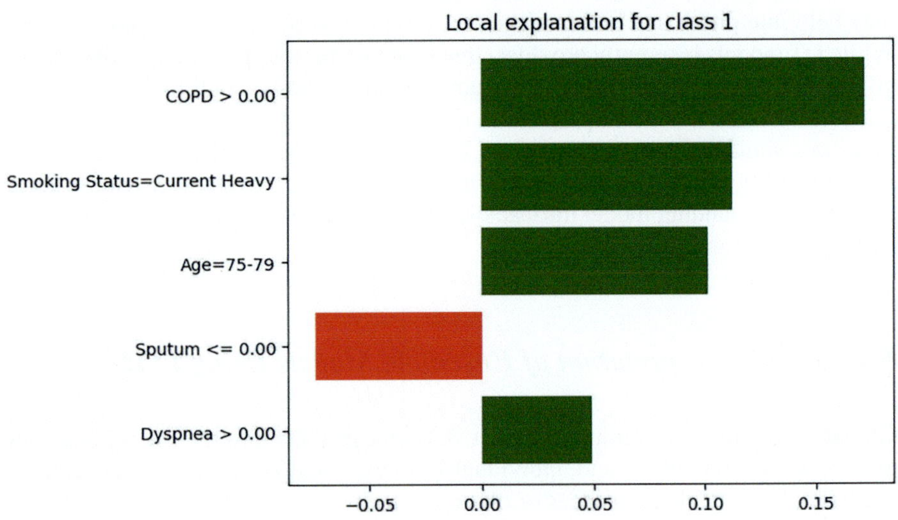

Fig. 7 Model prediction and actual outcome both positive for individual observation for RF

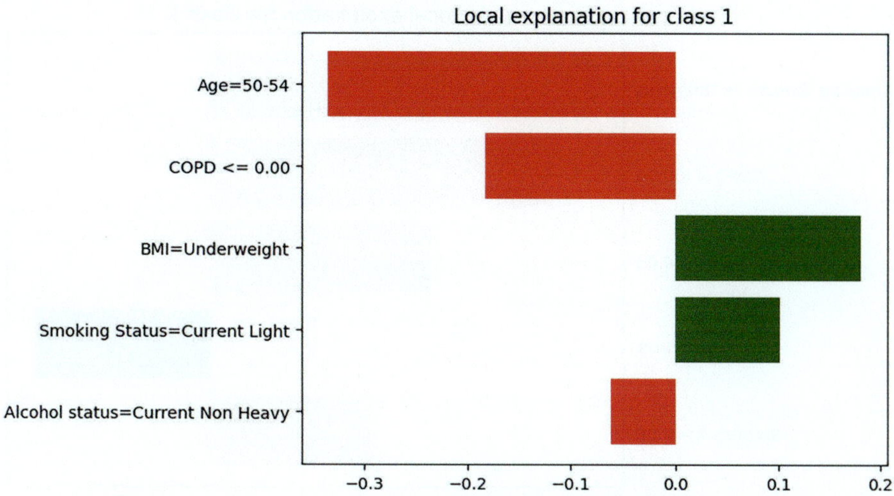

Fig. 8 Model prediction and actual outcome both negative for individual observation for XGB

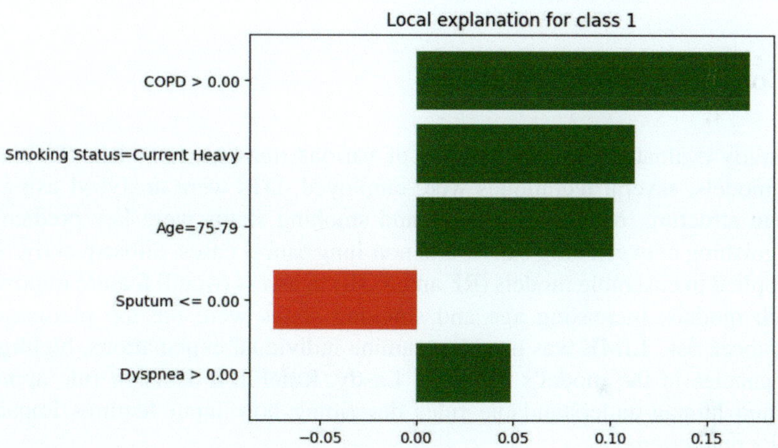

Fig. 9 Predicted positive, actual negative for RF model

By analyzing these factors, we can gain valuable insights into the model's behavior and potentially improve its accuracy.

Lastly, we will explore an observation where the XGB model predicted a negative outcome, but the actual outcome turned out to be positive depicted in Fig. 10. Despite the patient being in a higher age category, other factors played a crucial role. The absence of COPD, hemoptysis, and low smoking status collectively contributed to the negative prediction by the model. Therefore, examining individual-level explanations can provide valuable insights into the discrepancies in the model's behavior. Therefore, by understanding the specific factors that influence predictions, we can refine and enhance the model's accuracy.

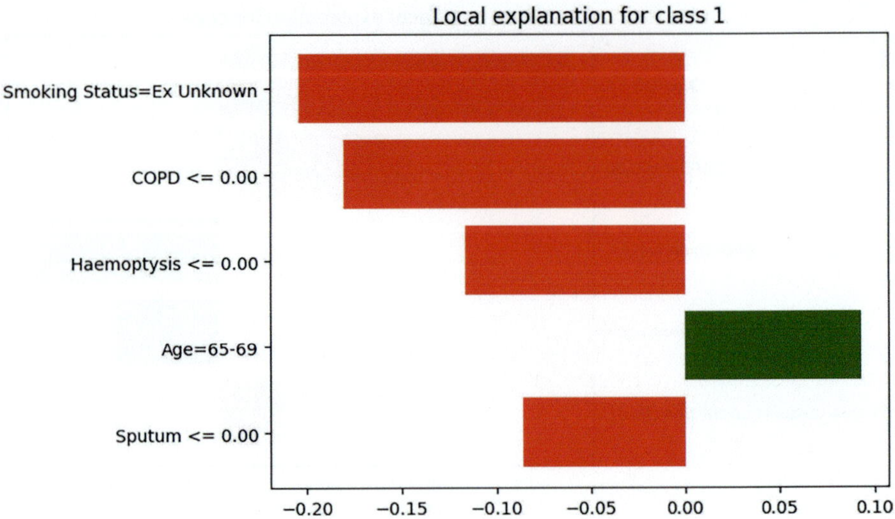

Fig. 10 Predicted negative, actual positive for XGB model

7 Conclusion and Discussion

This study evaluated the performance of various tree-based models. To interpret these models, several techniques were employed. DTs were analyzed using their inherent structure, revealing that age and smoking status were key predictors in distinguishing between lung cancer and non-lung cancer cases. Subsequently, SHAP was applied to ensemble models (RF and XGB) to assess overall feature importance. In both models, increasing age and smoking status were the top predictors for lung cancer risk. LIME was used to examine individual explanations, highlighting discrepancies in the model's behavior. Lastly, RuleFit, a decision rule approach, identified human-understandable rules describing how input features impact the model's predictions.

Acknowledgments This work is supported by UKRI through the Horizon Europe Guarantee Scheme (project number: 10078953) for the European Commission funded PHASE IV AI project (Grant Agreement No. 101095384) under the Horizon Europe Programme. Teena Rai is funded by the NTU VC PhD studentship.

References

1. Akil S, Sekkate S, Adib A. Interpretable credit scoring model via rule ensemble. In: International conference on advanced intelligent systems for sustainable development. Springer; 2022. pp 903–11.
2. Bach PB, Kattan MW, Thornquist MD, Kris MG, Tate RC, Barnett MJ, Hsieh LJ, Begg CB. Variations in lung cancer risk among smokers. J Natl Cancer Inst. 2003;95(6):470–8.

3. Bouchardy C, Benhamou S, Schaffar R, Verkooijen HM, Fioretta G, Schubert H, Vinh-Hung V, Soria JC, Vlastos G, Rapiti E. Lung cancer mortality risk among breast cancer patients treated with anti-estrogens. Cancer. 2011;117(6):1288–95.
4. Briggs E, de Kamps M, Hamilton W, Johnson O, McInerney CD, Neal RD. Machine learning for risk prediction of oesophago-gastric cancer in primary care: Comparison with existing risk-assessment tools. Cancers. 2022;14(20):5023.
5. Cancer Research UK. Lung cancer statistics. 2015. https://www.cancerresearchuk.org/health-professional/cancer-statistics/statistics-by-cancer-type/lung-cancer
6. Cassidy A, Myles JP, van Tongeren M, Page R, Liloglou T, Duffy S, Field J. The LLP risk model: An individual risk prediction model for lung cancer. Br J Cancer. 2008;98(2):270–6.
7. Cooley ME. Symptoms in adults with lung cancer: A systematic research review. J Pain Symptom Manag. 2000;19(2):137–53.
8. Durham AL, Adcock IM. The relationship between COPD and lung cancer. Lung Cancer. 2015;90(2):121–7.
9. Friedman JH, Popescu BE. Predictive learning via rule ensembles. Ann Appl Stat. 2008;2(3):916–54.
10. Gould MK, Huang BZ, Tammemagi MC, Kinar Y, Shiff R. Machine learning for early lung cancer identification using routine clinical and laboratory data. Am J Respir Crit Care Med. 2021;204(4):445–53.
11. Hastie T, Tibshirani R, Friedman JH, Friedman JH. The elements of statistical learning: Data mining, inference, and prediction, New York, Springer; 2009.
12. Herrett E, Gallagher AM, Bhaskaran K, Forbes H, Mathur R, Van Staa T, Smeeth L. Data resource profile: Clinical practice research datalink (CPRD). Int J Epidemiol. 2015;44(3):827–36.
13. Inskip PD, Stovall M, Flannery JT. Lung cancer risk and radiation dose among women treated for breast cancer. JNCI: J Natl Cancer Inst. 1994;86(13):983–8.
14. James G, Witten D, Hastie T, Tibshirani R, Taylor J. An introduction to statistical learning: With applications in python. Cham, Switzerland, Springer; 2023.
15. Katki HA, Kovalchik SA, Berg CD, Cheung LC, Chaturvedi AK. Development and validation of risk models to select ever-smokers for CT lung cancer screening. JAMA. 2016;315(21):2300–11.
16. Kobylińska K, Orłowski T, Adamek M, Biecek P. Explainable machine learning for lung cancer screening models. Appl Sci. 2022;12(4):1926.
17. de Koning HJ, van Der Aalst CM, de Jong PA, Scholten ET, Nackaerts K, Heuvelmans MA, Lammers JWJ, Weenink C, Yousaf-Khan U, Horeweg N, et al. Reduced lung-cancer mortality with volume CT screening in a randomized trial. N Eng J Med. 2020;382(6):503–13.
18. Liu XY, Wu J, Zhou ZH. Exploratory undersampling for class-imbalance learning. IEEE Trans Syst Man Cybern Part B (Cybern). 2008;39(2):539–50.
19. Lundberg SM, Lee SI. A unified approach to interpreting model predictions. In: Advances in neural information processing systems, vol 30. Curran Associates, Inc.; 2017, pp 4765–74.
20. Molnar C. Interpretable machine learning, 2nd edn.; 2022. https://christophm.github.io/interpretable-ml-book
21. Rai T, Shen Y, Kaur J, He J, Mahmud M, Brown DJ, Baldwin DR, O'Dowd E, Hubbard R. Decision tree approaches to select high risk patients for lung cancer screening based on the UK primary care data. In: Juarez JM, Marcos M, Stiglic G, Tucker A, editors. International conference on artificial intelligence in medicine. Lecture Notes in Computer Science, Springer; 2023. pp. 35–9.
22. Rai T, Shen Y, He J, Mahmud M, Brown DJ, Kaur J, O'Dowd E, Baldwin DR, Hubbard R. Understanding feature importance of prediction models based on lung cancer primary care data. In: 2024 International Joint Conference on Neural Networks (IJCNN); 2024. pp 1–8. doi:10.1109/IJCNN60899.2024.10650819

23. Raji OY, Duffy SW, Agbaje OF, Baker SG, Christiani DC, Cassidy A, Field JK. Predictive accuracy of the liverpool lung project risk model for stratifying patients for computed tomography screening for lung cancer: A case–control and cohort validation study. Ann Int Med. 2012;157(4):242–50.
24. Ribeiro MT, Singh S, Guestrin C. "Why should i trust you?" explaining the predictions of any classifier. In: Proceedings of the 22nd ACM SIGKDD international conference on knowledge discovery and data mining; 2016. pp 1135–44.
25. Tammemagi MC, Katki HA, Hocking WG, Church TR, Caporaso N, Kvale PA, Chaturvedi AK, Silvestri GA, Riley TL, Commins J, Berg CD. Selection criteria for lung-cancer screening. N Engl J Med. 2013;368(8):728–36.
26. Tammemägi MC, Ten Haaf K, Toumazis I, Kong CY, Han SS, Jeon J, Commins J, Riley T, Meza R. Development and validation of a multivariable lung cancer risk prediction model that includes low-dose computed tomography screening results: A secondary analysis of data from the national lung screening trial. JAMA Netw Open. 2019;2(3):e190204.
27. UK NSC. Lung cancer – UK National Screening Committee; 2024. https://view-health-screening-recommendations.service.gov.uk/lung-cancer

LIME and GraphLIME Coupled with a Features-Attention Mechanism for Thoracic Diagnosis Improvement

Darian M. Onchis, Flavia Costi, Codruta Istin, and Gabriel V. Cozma

Contents

Abstract This chapter explores the significant impact that explainability methods have within the clinical diagnosis field, focusing on how the advanced application of LIME and GraphLIME can enhance the predictability and performance of models.

These authors contributed equally to this work.

D. M. Onchis · F. Costi (✉)
Computer Science, West University of Timisoara, Timisoara, Timis, Romania
e-mail: darian.onchis@e-uvt.ro; flavia.costi@e-uvt.ro

C. Istin
Computer and Information Technology, Politehnica University, Traian Lalescu, Timisoara, Timis, Romania
e-mail: codruta.istin@upt.ro

G. V. Cozma
Thoracic Surgery, Victor Babes University of Medicine and Pharmacy, Timisoara, Timis, Romania
e-mail: gabriel.cozma@umft.ro

R. Ortale et al. (eds.), *Explainable Machine Intelligence in Healthcare*,
https://doi.org/10.1007/978-3-031-91379-2_7

We investigate how the extraction and analysis of relevant features through an attention mechanism directly influence the accuracy of predictions in diagnosing thoracic diseases. A clear distinction is made between LIME and GraphLIME, highlighting the advantages of each method and their applicability in the context of analyzing tabular datasets and images. By implementing these explainability techniques, the chapter demonstrates a notable improvement in model performance, achieving at least a 25% increase in accuracy, aided by the integration of attention mechanisms. The outcomes are illustrated through ROC curves, confusion matrices, and supplementary plots, providing a detailed insight into the mechanisms and architecture underlying the enhancement of predictions. This exploration emphasizes the importance of adopting explainability methods in thoracic diagnosis, suggesting that a deep understanding of data and the prediction process can lead to significant advancements in diagnostic precision. Additionally, this chapter proposes a new perspective on model interpretability, suggesting that such insights could pave the way for more personalized and effective medical treatments, further underscoring the potential of explainability in transforming healthcare analytics.

Keywords Neural networks · Deep supervised learning · Thoracic dataset · Explainability · Attention mechanism · Graph neural network

1 Introduction

This chapter proposes to integrate explainability as a feedback signal for the enhancement of neural networks, specifically targeting the diagnosis of thoracic issues. At the heart of our methodology lies the innovative application of feature attention, a technique designed to refine the model's focus on the most informative aspects of the data, thereby significantly improving its diagnostic capabilities. The cornerstone of our approach is the strategic utilization of explainability models, namely, GraphLIME and LIME, which serve as our primary tools for dissecting and understanding the model's predictions.

Based on the use of explainability methods, we aim to shed light on the intricate decision-making processes of neural networks, transforming this insight into a tangible improvement in performance. The chapter indicates the process of coupling the explainability signal with feature attention mechanisms, illustrating how this synergy not only enhances the model's accuracy but also its interpretability. This approach is particularly pertinent in the context of thoracic diseases, where the precision of diagnosis can have profound implications on patient outcomes [1].

We present the application of this method across various datasets pertaining to thoracic problems, demonstrating its versatility and effectiveness in different scenarios. Through a combination of theoretical exposition and practical examples, the chapter aims to equip the reader with a comprehensive understanding of how explainability signals, when effectively integrated with feature attention, can transform the field of medical diagnosis. By the end of this chapter, the reader will gain insight into the cutting-edge techniques that are setting new benchmarks in the accuracy and reliability of thoracic disease diagnostics, marking a significant step forward in the quest for more responsive and patient-centric healthcare solutions [2, 3].

2 Description of the LIME Algorithm and Its Applications

Our objective is to thoroughly investigate the architecture of LIME to discover ways to boost its effectiveness. LIME, renowned for its robustness and popularity, plays a pivotal role in the interpretability and explainability of complex models.

Our analysis will also include evaluating LIME's performance across various dataset types, including both tabular and image-based datasets. This holistic approach will enable us to evaluate LIME's versatility and adaptability in managing different data structures, an aspect for its application across multiple domains that demand high accuracy and interpretability.

Through this comprehensive analysis of both structured and unstructured data, we aim to identify insights that could lead to the creation of more sophisticated, efficient, and broadly applicable attention mechanisms. This effort seeks not only to enhance the capabilities of this widely used mechanism but also to contribute to future advancements in the field of machine learning interpretability and explainability [2].

2.1 Presentation of the LIME Algorithm

LIME is designed to improve the transparency and understandability of complex machine learning models. Its unique architecture and methodology enable it to generate explanations for the predictions of any model, regardless of its complexity, making it an invaluable tool for data scientists and researchers seeking to demystify model decisions [4].

2.1.1 Architecture

LIME's architecture is ingeniously simple yet profoundly effective in breaking down the decisions of complex models. The process begins with the recognition that while global interpretability may be challenging for highly intricate models, local interpretability is more feasible and equally valuable.

The first step in the LIME process involves creating perturbations of the input data. These perturbations are slight variations of the original data point, generated to create a neighborhood of data around the original point. This neighborhood helps in understanding how small changes in input can affect the model's predictions [4].

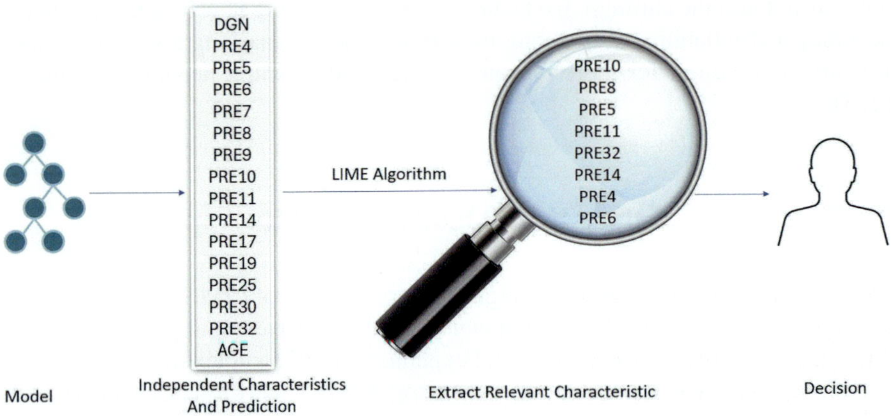

Fig. 1 LIME architecture for tabular dataset

Once the synthetic samples are generated, LIME assigns weights to these samples based on their proximity to the original input. This is typically done using a kernel function, such as an exponential kernel, which ensures that samples closer to the original input have more influence on the explanation model than those further away. This weighting is important as it reflects the local nature of the explanation, prioritizing information that is most relevant to the specific prediction being explained [5].

With the generated and weighted samples at hand, LIME proceeds to train a simple, interpretable model on this dataset. The choice of model is significant; it needs to be complex enough to capture the essential patterns in the data but simple enough to be inherently interpretable. Common choices include linear models for tabular data, decision trees, or even sparse linear models that focus on a subset of features for clarity (see Fig. 1).

The final step is the generation of explanations based on the parameters of the simple model trained in the previous step. For instance, in a linear model, the coefficients assigned to each feature can be interpreted as the importance of that feature in the model's prediction, within the local context of the input data point. These explanations provide insights into why the model made a specific prediction, highlighting the features that were most influential.

2.1.2 Benefits

The utilization of local interpretable model-agnostic explanations brings forth a suite of advantages that address some of the most challenging aspects of machine learning interpretability and trustworthiness. One of LIME's most pivotal attributes is its model agnosticism. This quality allows LIME to be applied across a vast array of machine learning models, irrespective of their complexity or the specifics of their internal workings. This universality not only provides practitioners with the flexibility in model selection and application but also ensures that LIME's benefits can be leveraged in a wide range of scenarios, from simple linear models to intricate deep learning architectures [6].

LIME enhances interpretability by creating simpler, local approximations of complex models around specific predictions. This approach translates the often opaque decision-making processes of sophisticated models into more human-readable and understandable terms. By doing so, LIME demystifies the "black box" nature of many algorithms, making the rationale behind specific predictions accessible and clear. This clarity is especially valuable when dealing with features and their roles in model predictions. LIME excels at identifying and highlighting the features that significantly influence a model's predictions, thus providing deep insights into the model's behavior and allowing for a better understanding of the factors driving the outcomes.

The aspect of trust and transparency cannot be overstated. In fields where the implications of model predictions are relevant, the transparency afforded by LIME is invaluable. It not only facilitates a deeper trust in machine learning models by making their operations more transparent. This transparency is relevant for gaining the confidence of end-users and stakeholders, particularly in sectors where accountability and clarity are paramount.

Lastly, LIME's utility as a diagnostic tool embodies a significant advantage. It aids in the identification and correction of biases or inaccuracies within models, thereby contributing to the development of more reliable and fair algorithms. By pinpointing the features that lead to particular predictions, LIME allows for an evaluation of whether these predictions are based on valid correlations or if they reflect biases in the data or model. This diagnostic capability helps not only in improving model accuracy but also in ensuring that models operate in an equitable and just manner [7].

2.1.3 Pseudocode for LIME Algorithm

In this part, we delve into the workings of the LIME algorithm. The essence of LIME lies in its capacity to create interpretable models that approximate the predictions of potentially opaque, intricate models for individual instances. The approach hinges on generating perturbations of the input data, weighting these perturbations to reflect their proximity to the original data point, and then fitting a simple, interpretable model to these weighted examples. The coefficients or structure of this simpler model provide insights into what features the original, complex model is using to make its predictions.

The process begins with the generation of a set of perturbed samples around a specific data point of interest. This is achieved by slightly altering the features of the input data to create variations, which helps in understanding how small changes can influence the model's predictions. These new samples are then weighted according to their similarity to the original data point, ensuring that those closer in the feature space have a greater influence on the explanation model.

A simple model is subsequently trained on this weighted, perturbed dataset. The choice of a simple model is very important; it needs to balance interpretability with the ability to capture the nuanced decision boundary of the complex model around the data point. Linear models, decision trees, or similar interpretable models are typically employed for this purpose. The final step involves interpreting the parameters of this simple model to extract explanations for the original model's predictions.

The following pseudocode outlines the LIME algorithm's workflow, capturing the sequence of steps from perturbation generation to explanation extraction. This structured presentation not only clarifies the algorithm's operational blueprint but also sets the stage for discussing its application and impact further [6].

Algorithm 1 LIME algorithm in pseudocode

```
procedure GenerateSamples(x, N)
    PerturbedSamples ← []
    for i ← 1 to N do
        Sample ← Perturb(x)
        PerturbedSamples.append(Sample)
    end for
    return PerturbedSamples
end procedure
procedure Perturb(x)
    // Implementation depends on data type
    return perturbed_x
end procedure
procedure ComputeProximity(x, PerturbedSamples)
    Weights ← []
    for Sample in PerturbedSamples do
        Weight ← SimilarityFunction(x, Sample)
        Weights.append(Weight)
    end for
    return Weights
end procedure
procedure TrainLocalModel(PerturbedSamples, Weights, M)
    Labels ← M.predict(PerturbedSamples)
    LocalModel ← TrainSimpleModel(PerturbedSamples, Labels, Weights)
    return LocalModel
end procedure
PerturbedSamples ← GenerateSamples(x, N)
Weights ← ComputeProximity(x, PerturbedSamples)
LocalModel ← TrainLocalModel(PerturbedSamples, Weights, M)
Explanation ← ExtractFeatureImportance(LocalModel)
return Explanation
```

3 Description of the GraphLIME Algorithm and Its Applications

In this section, we are dedicated to advancing our understanding of GraphLIME, a variant less explored than its counterpart, LIME. Our observation into the intricacies of GraphLIME will not only involve an analysis of its performance. By dissecting the architecture of GraphLIME, we aim to uncover the layers that might hold the key to enhancing its efficacy. This exploration is motivated by the recognition that, despite its foundational status, GraphLIME remains underutilized and somewhat overshadowed by the more widely recognized LIME, presenting an opportunity for discovery and optimization.

Our investigation will be guided by several core objectives: to elucidate the specific components and operations that distinguish GraphLIME, to evaluate its performance across various datasets and contexts, and to identify any potential areas where its standard implementation may fall short. This endeavor is not just about benchmarking GraphLIME against established metrics; it's about pushing the boundaries of what this mechanism can achieve. By pinpointing where and how GraphLIME's performance can be augmented, we open the door to making it not just a viable alternative to LIME but possibly a preferred solution in scenarios where its unique capabilities can be fully leveraged.

Given its lesser-known status, a significant part of our discussion will also be relevant, aiming to illuminate the principles behind GraphLIME's methodology. This includes an examination of how GraphLIME processes and interprets data, particularly graph-based data, which stands at the heart of its innovative approach [2].

This section want to not only foster a deeper appreciation of GraphLIME's potential but also to catalyze further research and application of this attention mechanism. Through this comprehensive analysis, we seek to lay the groundwork for future innovations that could extend the frontier of explainability in machine learning, making sophisticated models more accessible, interpretable, and, importantly, more effective in addressing real-world problems [8].

3.1 *Presentation of the GraphLIME Algorithm*

GraphLIME, an innovative extension of LIME, represents a significant advancement in the interpretability of machine learning models, especially those applied to graph data. As complex data structures like graphs become increasingly prevalent in various fields, including biomedical research, the ability to explain model predictions transparently becomes necessary. This detailed examination of GraphLIME delves into its architecture, benefits, and applications, particularly in the biomedical domain, highlighting its importance.

3.1.1 Architecture

The architecture of GraphLIME is a framework designed to address the unique challenges of interpreting machine learning models that operate on graph data. This deep dive into its architecture reveals the meticulous considerations and innovative solutions that make GraphLIME particularly effective for graph-based applications.

GraphLIME's architecture can be broken down into several components, each contributing to its ability to generate local, interpretable explanations for graph data.

The initial step in the GraphLIME process involves identifying the neighborhood for a target node. This neighborhood consists of nodes directly connected to the target node, reflecting the local structure and features relevant to the target. This localization is important in graph data, where the global structure might be too complex for effective interpretation. The method for neighborhood selection is carefully designed to balance comprehensiveness with computational efficiency, ensuring that the neighborhood is sufficiently representative but not overly broad.

Once the neighborhood is identified, GraphLIME focuses on representing the features of this localized area in a manner conducive to interpretable modeling. This involves extracting and possibly transforming the features of the nodes within the neighborhood to form a feature space that can be analyzed. Given the diversity of graph data, from simple node attributes to complex relational features, this step is vital for ensuring that the subsequent explanation is grounded in the actual data structure.

A standout feature of GraphLIME's architecture is the integration of the Hilbert-Schmidt Independence Criterion Lasso method for feature selection. Unlike traditional linear feature selection methods, HSIC Lasso can capture nonlinear dependencies between features and the prediction. This capability is particularly important in graph data, where the relationships between nodes and features may not be linear. By applying HSIC Lasso, GraphLIME selects a subset of features from the node's neighborhood that have the most significant impact on the model's prediction, ensuring that the explanation focuses on the most relevant information [9].

With the relevant features identified, GraphLIME proceeds to train a simple, interpretable model on the data from the target node's neighborhood. This model, often a linear model or decision tree, is designed to mimic the prediction behavior of the complex model for the target node, based solely on the selected features. The simplicity of this model is key to its interpretability, as it allows for straightforward understanding of how each feature influences the prediction.

The important part of the GraphLIME process is the generation of explanations. These explanations are derived from the simple model's parameters, such as the weights or splits, which directly correlate to the importance of each selected feature. By interpreting these parameters, GraphLIME provides insights into why the complex model made a specific prediction for the target node, grounded in the local context of the node's neighborhood (see Fig. 2 for more details) [8].

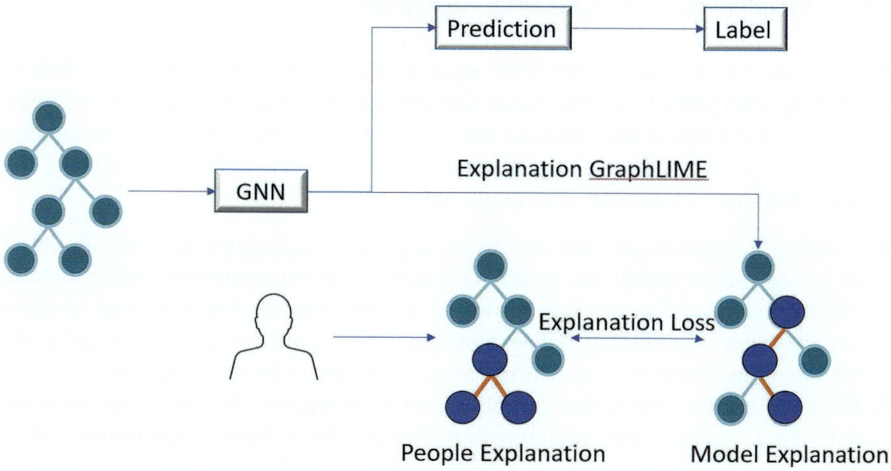

Fig. 2 GraphLIME architecture for tabular dataset

3.1.2 Benefits

GraphLIME stands out as an innovative approach to demystifying the predictions of machine learning models trained on graph data, offering several compelling advantages that cater to the growing demand for transparency and interpretability in AI systems. Primarily, its model-agnostic nature ensures broad applicability across a variety of models, making it a versatile tool for diverse applications. Unlike traditional interpretation methods, which may struggle with the intricate structures inherent in graph data, GraphLIME is specifically designed to navigate these complexities, providing clear, localized explanations that focus on individual nodes within a graph. This node-centric perspective is invaluable, especially in fields like biomedicine, where understanding the role and influence of specific entities (e.g., genes, proteins) within a network can lead to significant insights. Furthermore, the use of HSIC Lasso for feature selection allows GraphLIME to capture and highlight nonlinear dependencies between features and predictions, offering a nuanced understanding of the model's decision-making process. By generating interpretable explanations even from highly complex models, GraphLIME enhances trust in AI applications, fostering greater confidence among users and stakeholders [2]. Its ability to elucidate the reasons behind a model's predictions not only aids in validating the model's reliability but also opens up opportunities for identifying potential areas for model improvement, contributing to the development of more accurate and robust AI systems.

3.1.3 Pseudocode for GraphLIME Algorithm

The pseudocode for the GraphLIME algorithm presents a structured approach to generating interpretable explanations for predictions made by machine learning models on graph-based data, particularly focusing on the explanations for individual nodes. The process encapsulates several key steps, each tailored to address the unique challenges of dealing with graph data:

1. Identify Neighborhood: The algorithm begins by identifying the neighborhood of a target node within the graph. This neighborhood comprises nodes that are directly connected to or in proximity to the target node. The selection of these nodes is very important as it determines the local context around the target node, which is fundamental to generating an accurate and relevant explanation.
2. Extract Features: Once the neighborhood is identified, the next step involves extracting (and possibly transforming) features from these neighboring nodes. This step is designed to compile a comprehensive set of features that represent the local structure and characteristics of the graph around the target node, forming a feature matrix that encapsulates the local information.
3. Generate Synthetic Data: With the feature matrix ready, the algorithm then generates synthetic data based on these features. This synthetic dataset aims to mimic the variations in the neighborhood's feature space, providing a basis for training a local, interpretable model that can approximate the original complex model's predictions.
4. HSIC Lasso Feature Selection: A step in the process is the application of the Hilbert-Schmidt Independence Criterion Lasso method for feature selection. This nonlinear feature selection technique is adept at identifying the subset of features from the synthetic dataset that are most influential for the prediction of the target node. This step ensures that the explanation focuses on the most relevant features, enhancing the interpretability of the final explanation.
5. Train Local Model: With the most relevant features selected, the algorithm proceeds to train a simple, interpretable model on this refined dataset. This model is trained specifically to mimic the original complex model's prediction behavior for the target node, based on the locally relevant features. The simplicity of this model is key to ensuring that the explanations generated are understandable and accessible.
6. Generate Explanation: The final step involves analyzing the trained local model to determine the importance of each selected feature in influencing the model's prediction for the target node. This analysis yields an explanation that highlights the key features and their contributions, providing insights into the rationale behind the complex model's prediction [2].

Algorithm 2 GraphLIME algorithm in pseudocode

Require: Graph G, target node n, model M, number of samples N
Ensure: Explanation E for the prediction of node n

```
function IDENTIFYNEIGHBORHOOD(G, n)
    Determine the neighborhood of n in G
    return neighborhood
end function
function EXTRACTFEATURES(neighborhood)
    Extract and/or transform features for each node in the neighborhood
    return feature matrix X
end function
function GENERATESYNTHETICDATA(X, N)
    Generate N synthetic samples based on the feature matrix X
    return synthetic dataset X'
end function
function HSICLASSOSELECTION(X', M, n)
    Apply HSIC Lasso to select most relevant features for n's prediction
    return selected features X''
end function
function TRAINLOCALMODEL(X'', M)
    Train a simple model on X'' to approximate M's behavior near n
    return local model L
end function
function GENERATEEXPLANATION(L)
    Analyze L to determine feature importance for n's prediction
    return explanation E based on feature importance
end function
neighborhood ← IDENTIFYNEIGHBORHOOD(G, n)
X ← EXTRACTFEATURES(neighborhood)
X' ← GENERATESYNTHETICDATA(X, N)
X'' ← HSICLASSOSELECTION(X', M, n)
L ← TRAINLOCALMODEL(X'', M)
E ← GENERATEEXPLANATION(L)
return E
```

4 Presentation of the Datasets

The Thoracic Surgery dataset, available on Kaggle, represents a rich collection of clinical data focused on patients undergoing thoracic surgery. Sourced from a reputable platform for data science competitions and research, Kaggle, this dataset offers a comprehensive insight into the myriad factors influencing surgical outcomes and patient recovery. It encompasses a broad spectrum of preoperative conditions, demographic details, and postoperative survival indicators, structured to facilitate in-depth analysis and predictive modeling in medical research. The dataset comprises 17 features, of which 16 are independent variables representing factors that lead to thoracic issues, and 1 dependent variable that encompasses the outcome: whether the patient suffers from thoracic problems or not. The dataset is meticulously organized, with each row representing a patient case and the following attributes captured to detail the preoperative and postoperative scenario:

- Diagnosis (DGN): The categorical variable for diagnosis clarifies the nature of thoracic diseases treated, ranging from various lung conditions to other diseases affecting the thoracic cavity. The dataset categorizes these conditions into distinct classifications such as DGN2, DGN3, etc., enabling researchers to analyze disease-specific outcomes and trends.
- Forced Vital Capacity (PRE4) and Volume Exhaled (PRE5): These pulmonary function tests quantify lung capacity and function through measured air volumes expelled during forced breathing exercises. The variables are essential for evaluating respiratory health pre-surgery and can significantly impact surgical planning and prognosis.
- Performance Status (PRE6): Utilizing codes like PRZ0, PRZ1, and PRZ2, this attribute assesses a patient's physical health and daily activity capabilities. A pivotal preoperative indicator, it helps gauge the patient's resilience and potential for postoperative recovery.
- Symptom and Risk Factor Indicators (PRE7–PRE11, PRE14, PRE17, PRE19, PRE25, PRE30, PRE32): These binary variables provide a snapshot of the patient's health status by marking the presence or absence of specific symptoms and conditions (e.g., cough, diabetes). This detailed symptomatology and risk profiling are relevant for personalized patient management strategies.
- Age (AGE): Patient age, a vital demographic variable, influences the surgical approach, risk assessment, and recovery expectations, providing a foundational context for outcome analysis.
- One-Year Mortality Risk (Risk1Yr): Perhaps one of the most important attributes, this binary outcome variable predicts the likelihood of patient mortality within a year post-surgery. It is a key metric for evaluating surgical success and long-term efficacy [10].

As can be observed in Fig. 3, there is a discrepancy between the number of patients suffering from this disease and those who are not. Four hundred patients are healthy, yet almost 100 have thoracic issues.

The values that the independent variables can take are as follows:

- DGN: Categorical variable indicating the type of thoracic disease diagnosed in the patient.
- PRE4: A numerical variable representing the volume of air that the patient can forcibly exhale from the lungs after taking the deepest breath possible.
- PRE5: A numerical variable indicating the volume of air expelled during the first second of a forceful exhalation.
- PRE6: Categorical variable indicating the patient's overall health and ability to perform daily activities, coded with specific statuses like PRZ0, PRZ1, and PRZ2.
- PRE7: Binary variable indicating the presence (T) or absence (F) of pain before surgery.

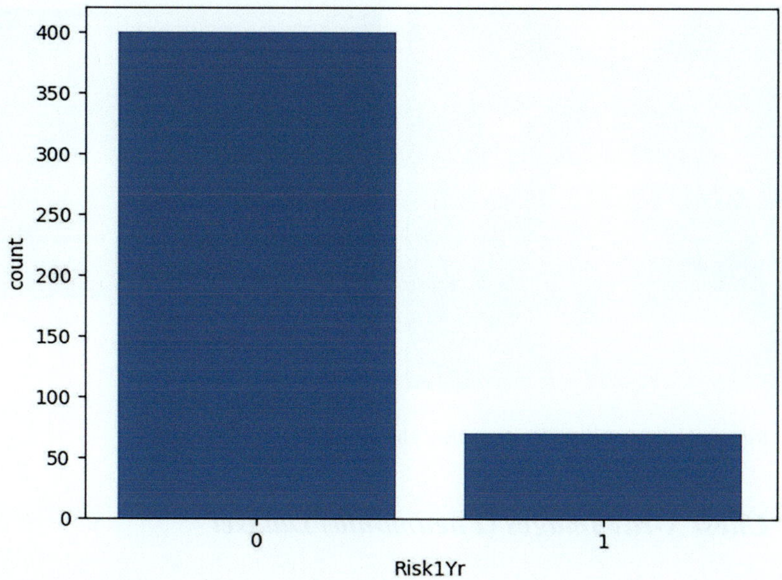

Fig. 3 Representation of Risk1Yr-dependent characteristic

- PRE8: Binary variable indicating the presence (T) or absence (F) of coughing up blood before surgery.
- PRE9: Binary variable indicating the presence (T) or absence (F) of difficulty breathing before surgery.
- PRE10: Binary variable indicating the presence (T) or absence (F) of cough before surgery.
- PRE11: Binary variable indicating the presence (T) or absence (F) of generalized weakness before surgery.
- PRE14: Indicates the size or direct extent of the primary tumor, with various categorical levels.
- PRE17: Binary variable indicating the presence (T) or absence (F) of type 2 diabetes mellitus.
- PRE19: Binary variable indicating the presence (T) or absence (F) of myocardial infarction (heart attack) up to 6 months before surgery.
- PRE25: Binary variable indicating the presence (T) or absence (F) of peripheral arterial diseases.
- PRE30: Binary variable indicating if the patient is a smoker (T) or not (F).
- PRE32: Binary variable indicating the presence (T) or absence (F) of asthma.
- AGE: Numerical variable indicating the age of the patient [11].

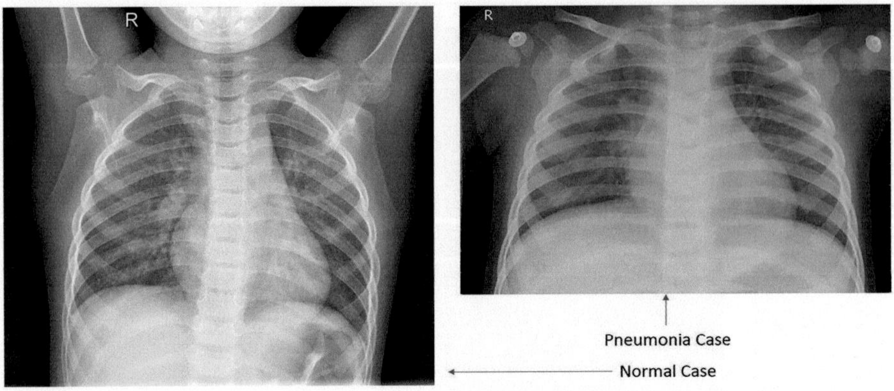

Fig. 4 Representation of Risk1Yr-dependent characteristic

4.1 Chest X-ray Images (Pneumonia) Dataset

The Chest X-ray Images (Pneumonia) dataset on Kaggle is a collection of chest radiograph images specifically assembled to aid in the development of automated diagnostic tools for pneumonia. It encompasses a comprehensive set of images divided into categories indicating the presence or absence of pneumonia. This resource is especially valuable for those in the fields of medical imaging and machine learning, providing a basis for training algorithms to differentiate between normal and pathological chest X-rays with the goal of enhancing diagnostic accuracy [12] (Fig. 4).

5 Application of LIME and GraphLIME to Medical Data

5.1 Applying LIME to Tabular Data

Explainability techniques have garnered significant attention for their role in unraveling the decision-making processes of complex models. Among these techniques, LIME stands out for its capacity to provide insights into model predictions on a per-instance basis. This chapter delves into the application of LIME on a tabular dataset, delineating the methodical approach undertaken to enhance the interpretability of a predictive model.

The initial was the selection of an optimal classifier for our dataset. The inherent characteristics of the dataset made it particularly amenable to classification algorithms. Among various classifiers evaluated, logistic regression was chosen for its suitability. This decision was predicated on several pivotal factors.

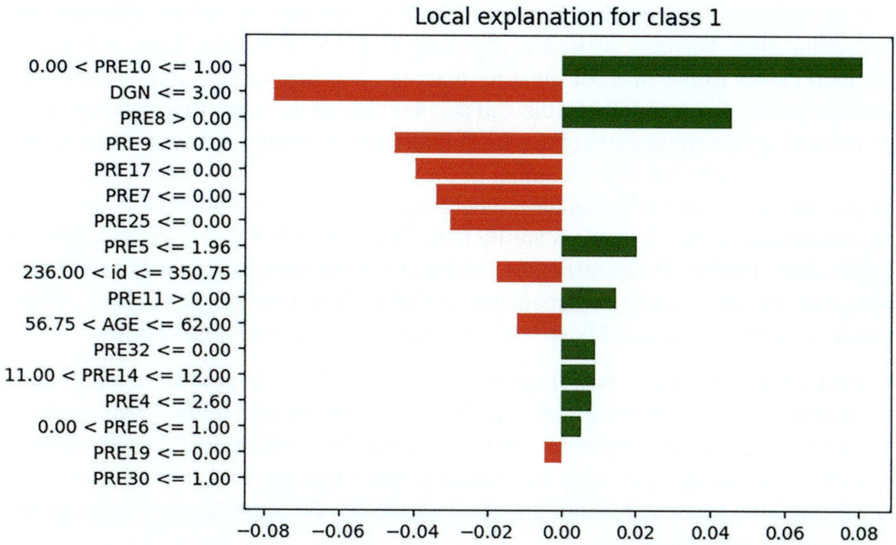

Fig. 5 Illustrative visualization of feature impact through LIME analysis

Firstly, logistic regression's inherent simplicity and transparency make it an exemplary model for interpretability. Unlike more complex models that operate as "black boxes," logistic regression provides clear insights into how each feature influences the outcome. Furthermore, its efficiency in handling binary outcomes, coupled with its robustness to small sample sizes and its ability to provide probabilities alongside predictions, renders it an ideal choice for datasets with binary dependent variables.

Following the application of the logistic regression classifier, the LIME technique was employed to shed light on the model's predictions. LIME operates by approximating the local decision boundary of the model around a given prediction, using a simpler model that is easier to interpret, such as a linear model. This approach allows us to dissect and understand the contribution of each feature to the prediction of a particular instance [13] (Fig. 5).

The illustrative figure below encapsulates the essence of LIME's explanatory power. Through this visualization, we can discern the impact of individual features on the dependent variable, Risk1Yr, post-model training. The graph elucidates which features positively or negatively influence the risk prediction, thereby offering a nuanced understanding of the model's behavior. For instance, if a feature is shown to significantly increase the risk, this insight can inform clinicians and patients alike about potential risk factors in clinical decision-making.

This application of LIME not only illuminates the model's predictive dynamics but also paves the way for more transparent and trustworthy AI solutions in healthcare. By demystifying the influence of specific features on predictions, we foster a collaborative environment where machine learning models can be assessed and improved upon, ensuring that the technology we rely on is both effective and understandable. Through such meticulous applications of explainability techniques, we inch closer to the ideal of creating machine learning models that are not only predictive but also comprehensible and accountable to the users they serve [14].

Following the application of the local interpretable model-agnostic explanations method to enhance our understanding of the logistic regression model's predictions on the dataset, several features have emerged as particularly influential in determining the outcome. These features are PRE10, PRE8, PRE5, PRE11, PRE32, PRE14, PRE4, and PRE6. Their relevance underscores the nuanced interplay between different variables and the dependent variable, Risk1Yr, in our dataset. These features have been grouped based on their apparent roles and implications:

- **PRE10 and PRE8:** These features are likely related to specific clinical measurements or patient characteristics. Their significant role in the LIME analysis suggests they hold substantial predictive value for the outcome. For example, if *PRE10* is a measure of lung function and *PRE8* pertains to a patient's age or the severity of a particular symptom, this underscores the importance of these factors in assessing surgical risks.
- **PRE5, PRE11, and PRE32:** This group of features probably encapsulates vital health indicators or demographic details. Their marked significance indicates the multifaceted nature of risk in thoracic surgeries. Comprehending the impact of these features can be pivotal in devising more refined preoperative evaluations and crafting personalized care strategies.
- **PRE14, PRE4, and PRE6:** These attributes may include further clinical parameters, historical health data, or lifestyle determinants that influence the surgical outcome. Their prominence in the LIME analysis underscores the myriad of factors that need consideration for accurate prediction and effective management of patient risk.

The identification of these relevant features through LIME's explainability technique provides valuable insights into the model's decision-making process. It allows healthcare professionals to focus on specific aspects of patient care and preoperative evaluation that are most indicative of surgical outcomes. For example, if certain features relate to modifiable risk factors, interventions could be designed to address these before surgery.

Moreover, the insight into feature relevance has broader implications for model development and refinement. Knowing which features significantly impact the model's predictions can guide further data collection and feature engineering efforts. It can also prompt researchers to investigate the underlying reasons why these features play an important role, potentially uncovering new clinical insights or reinforcing existing medical knowledge.

5.2 Applying LIME to Images

The Residual Network (ResNet) architecture [15] was employed as baseline for our experiments. Opting for the ResNet-18 model, characterized by its depth of 18 layers, our decision leaned on the model's proven track record in medical image classification capabilities.

To align the ResNet-18 architecture with our project's objectives, we meticulously customized its architecture. The modification was centered on the model's last layer, a fully connected layer, where we adjusted the output parameters to categorize images into two distinct classifications: "Normal" and "Pneumonia." This adjustment was relevant for the model to accurately address our binary classification challenge.

When the LIME algorithm is applied together with the ResNet-18 architecture for the analysis and interpretation of images, it significantly enhances the transparency and understanding of the model's decisions in image recognition tasks. The integration of LIME with ResNet-18, a deep and efficient model for image classification, reveals how various regions of an image contribute to the final classification, illuminating the often perceived "black box" process.

ResNet-18, being a convolutional neural network model with 18 layers, is frequently chosen for small image classification tasks due to its ability to learn complex features and its high performance. In the context of applying LIME, ResNet-18 is utilized to classify images, and LIME is applied to interpret and explain these classifications.

To generate interpretable explanations with LIME, the first step involves segmenting the image processed by ResNet-18 into superpixels, which are clusters of pixels with similar visual properties. This segmentation simplifies the image, making it easier to analyze. LIME then perturbs this image by randomly modifying the superpixels, turning different regions on or off, and observes how these changes affect the classification made by ResNet-18.

By assessing the impact of each perturbation on the classification, LIME can determine the importance of each superpixel to the model's prediction. This is achieved by training a simple model, such as a linear model, which approximates how the local features (superpixels) influence the final decision of the ResNet-18 model. The simple model, due to its interpretable nature, provides valuable insights into which regions of the image and what types of features lead to the specific classification of an image.

The advantage of combining LIME with ResNet-18 is the ability to see and understand which parts of an image are most relevant to the model's decision. This is important in fields such as medical imaging diagnostics, where understanding specific areas of a radiological image that indicate the presence of a condition can improve both the accuracy of diagnoses and practitioners' confidence in using machine learning technology. The explainability provided by LIME can aid in improving the model by identifying and correcting biases or classification errors. A primary outcome of applying LIME to images can be observed in Fig. 6 [15].

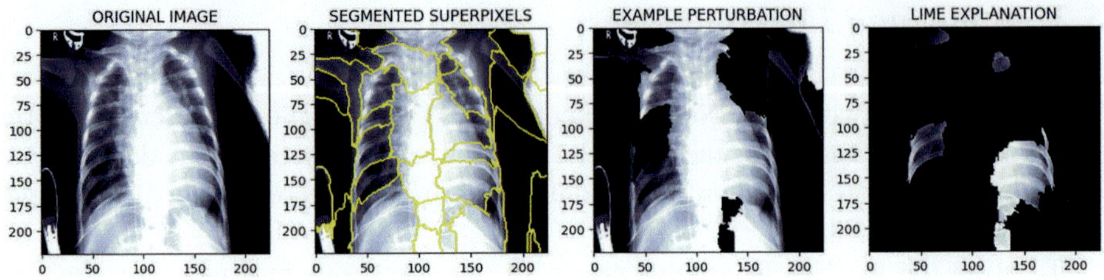

Fig. 6 LIME explanation for image dataset

5.3 *Applying GraphLIME to Tabular Data*

In this subsection, we delve into the application of the GraphLIME method, an advanced technique in the realm of explainable AI, tailored specifically to shed light on the nuances of tabular datasets. Our narrative unfolds through several meticulously orchestrated steps, beginning with the selection of an optimal model, transitioning through the intricacies of model architecture and training and culminating in the generation of perturbed samples to pierce the veil of model decisions.

At the outset, the pivotal task was to identify the most suitable machine learning model that could gracefully navigate the complexities of our dataset. After a comprehensive evaluation of various architectures, we settled on the sequential model. This choice was not arbitrary; the sequential model, renowned for its flexibility and efficiency, serves as an excellent foundation for both simple and complex neural network structures. The architecture we embraced for this endeavor was meticulously crafted, consisting of:

- A dense layer with 64 neurons, employing the "relu" activation function, taking the shape of our training data as its input dimension. This layer serves as the gateway, transforming the input data into a higher-dimensional space where nonlinear relationships can be discerned.
- Another dense layer, this time with 32 neurons, also utilizing the "relu" activation function. This layer further refines the representations learned by the previous layer, distilling the data into more abstract features.
- A final dense layer comprising a single neuron with a "sigmoid" activation function. This layer acts as the culmination of our model, distilling the complex relationships and patterns discovered in the data into a binary prediction.

With the architecture defined, we embarked on the training phase. This phase is not merely about adjusting weights and biases; it is a delicate dance of optimization, where the model learns from the data, improving its predictions with each iteration. We nourished our model with the dataset, allowing it to learn the subtle cues and patterns that define the outcome. The essence of GraphLIME lies in its ability to generate perturbed samples – variations of the original data that help illuminate the model's decision-making process. By carefully altering the data and observing the

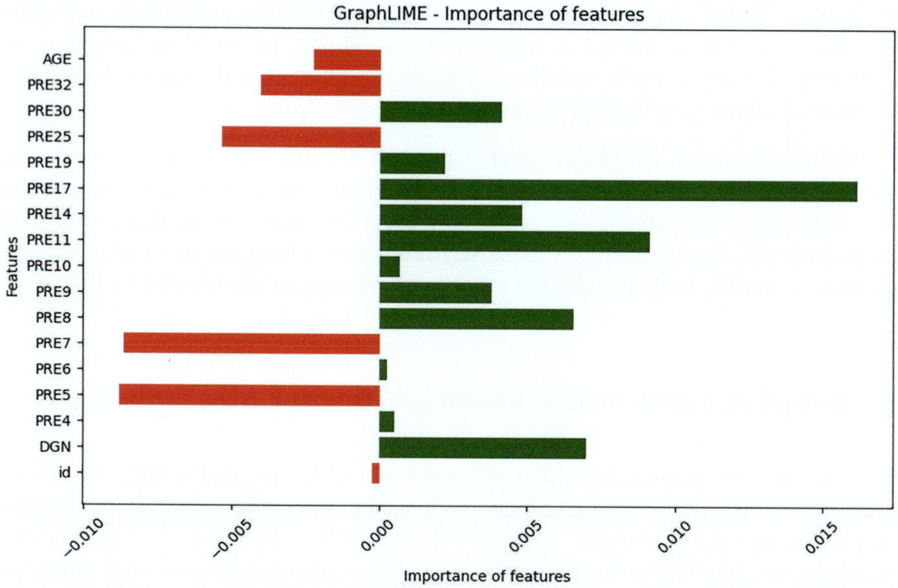

Fig. 7 Illustrative visualization of feature impact through GraphLIME analysis

model's reactions, we gain insights into which features wield the most influence and how they interact to shape the model's predictions (Fig. 7).

Utilizing GraphLIME to interpret a tabular dataset, particularly in healthcare, involves identifying key features that influence model predictions. This process has highlighted several features within a dataset aimed at predicting outcomes in thoracic surgery. The significant features are DGN, PRE4, PRE6, PRE8, PRE9, PRE10, PRE11, PRE14, PRE17, PRE19, and PRE30. Understanding the relevance of these features can greatly enhance decision-making processes in clinical settings:

- DGN: Represents the diagnosis, indicating the type of disease or condition. The diagnosis is fundamental in assessing the necessity of surgery and potential risks involved.
- PRE4 (Forced Vital Capacity, FVC) and PRE6 (Forced Expiratory Volume in One Second, FEV1): These are measures of lung function. High values typically indicate better lung performance, which is relevant for surgery candidates, especially in procedures involving the thorax.
- PRE8, PRE9, and PRE10: Although not specified, features like these could relate to other clinical measurements or patient-reported symptoms. Their significance suggests they play a role in evaluating surgical risk or patient outcomes.
- PRE11 (Pain): The presence of pain can indicate the severity and progression of a condition, influencing both the urgency and approach to surgery.
- PRE14 (Tumor Size): Directly correlates with cancer staging. Larger tumors might require more extensive surgical intervention and can impact prognosis.

- PRE17, PRE19, and PRE30: These features, while not detailed, likely represent additional clinical indicators such as comorbidities, patient demographics, or treatment history. Their influence on model predictions underscores the importance of a holistic patient assessment.

The identification of these features through GraphLIME sheds light on the complex factors that influence surgical outcomes and risks. This insight is important for healthcare professionals as it supports a more informed and nuanced approach to patient care. By focusing on these key predictors, clinicians can better stratify patients according to their risks and tailor interventions more effectively [16].

6 Coupling LIME with a Features-Attention Mechanism

The attention mechanism in neural networks is a technique that mimics cognitive attention by focusing on specific parts of the input data when making predictions or processing information [3]. It's particularly useful in the prediction of thoracic problems because it allows the model to pay more attention to relevant features in chest X-ray images or tabular data that may indicate the presence of conditions such as pneumonia (see Fig. 8).

We designed an attention mechanism consisting of three layers. The first two layers use the ReLU (Rectified Linear Unit) activation function, which helps in introducing nonlinearity to the model, allowing it to learn complex patterns by activating only positive inputs and setting negative values to zero. The final layer utilizes the sigmoid activation function, which outputs values between 0 and 1, making it suitable for binary classification tasks like identifying whether thoracic issues are present.

The combination of ReLU and sigmoid functions in an attention mechanism facilitates efficient feature learning and decision-making for both tabular and image datasets in thoracic problem detection, enhancing model accuracy by focusing on the most informative parts of the data.

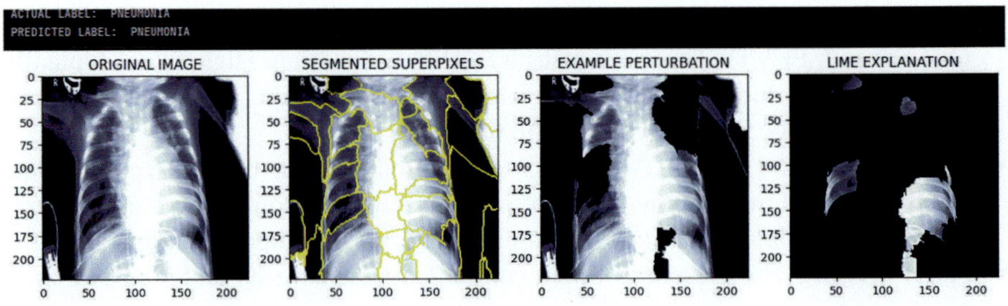

Fig. 8 Result after applying LIME and features-attention mechanism

Through the implementation of this attention mechanism, our goal is to synergize the aspects of explainability and focused attention to achieve a highly accurate prediction. This approach involves the integration of feature extraction with model enhancement via feature attention, leading to a remarkable improvement in prediction accuracy by more than 35%. By selectively applying the attention mechanism to essential features, we've managed to disregard less impactful variables, concentrating solely on those that significantly affect the model's outcome.

The application of this technique has yielded exceptionally positive results for both tabular datasets and images. The model's performance notably excels with image data, where the initial prediction accuracy of approximately 74% dramatically increased to over 98% following the implementation of LIME and the attention mechanism. This significant improvement highlights the technique's effectiveness in enhancing predictive accuracy across different types of data. Similarly, the technique has significantly enhanced performance with image datasets, increasing the accuracy from approximately 80% to over 96%. This improvement further demonstrates the method's capability in boosting prediction accuracy across diverse data types. These outcomes can be visualized and analyzed through ROC curves (receiver operating characteristic curve) and confusion matrices, providing a clear and comprehensive view of the model's performance improvements. The ROC curve is a graph that illustrates the diagnostic ability of a binary classifier system as its discrimination threshold is varied, by plotting the true positive rate (TPR) against the false positive rate (FPR) at various threshold settings. The confusion matrix, on the other hand, is a table used to describe the performance of a classification model on a set of test data for which the true values are known. It shows the actual versus predicted classifications and breaks down the results into true positives, false positives, true negatives, and false negatives, providing insight into any classification errors the model is making [17].

In the case of the tabular dataset, as depicted in Fig. 9, the ROC curve significantly approaches closer to 1 after applying the presented technique, indicating a substantial improvement in model specificity and sensitivity. The performance of the model is clearly visible to the naked eye by analyzing the figures below and comparing the two ROC curves.

Our exploratory phase kicked off with the application of the pretrained ResNet-18 model directly on a dataset comprised of chest X-ray images, categorizing them into "Normal" and "Pneumonia" without additional training. This preliminary trial yielded a notable accuracy rate of 74.29% and an ROC curve AUC of 0.52, demonstrating a modest advantage over random classification predictions.

To further refine our model's performance, we employed the LIME method. This approach was instrumental in pinpointing the features within the chest X-ray images that were most indicative of our categories of interest. Armed with this insight, we enhanced the ResNet-18 model by incorporating an attention mechanism, focusing the subsequent training phase – extended over 100 epochs – on these key features.

The adoption of this focused approach marked a significant leap in our model's accuracy, achieving an impressive rate of 98.312% and an ROC curve AUC of 0.99 (see Fig. 10). These outcomes not only reflect the effectiveness of precise feature

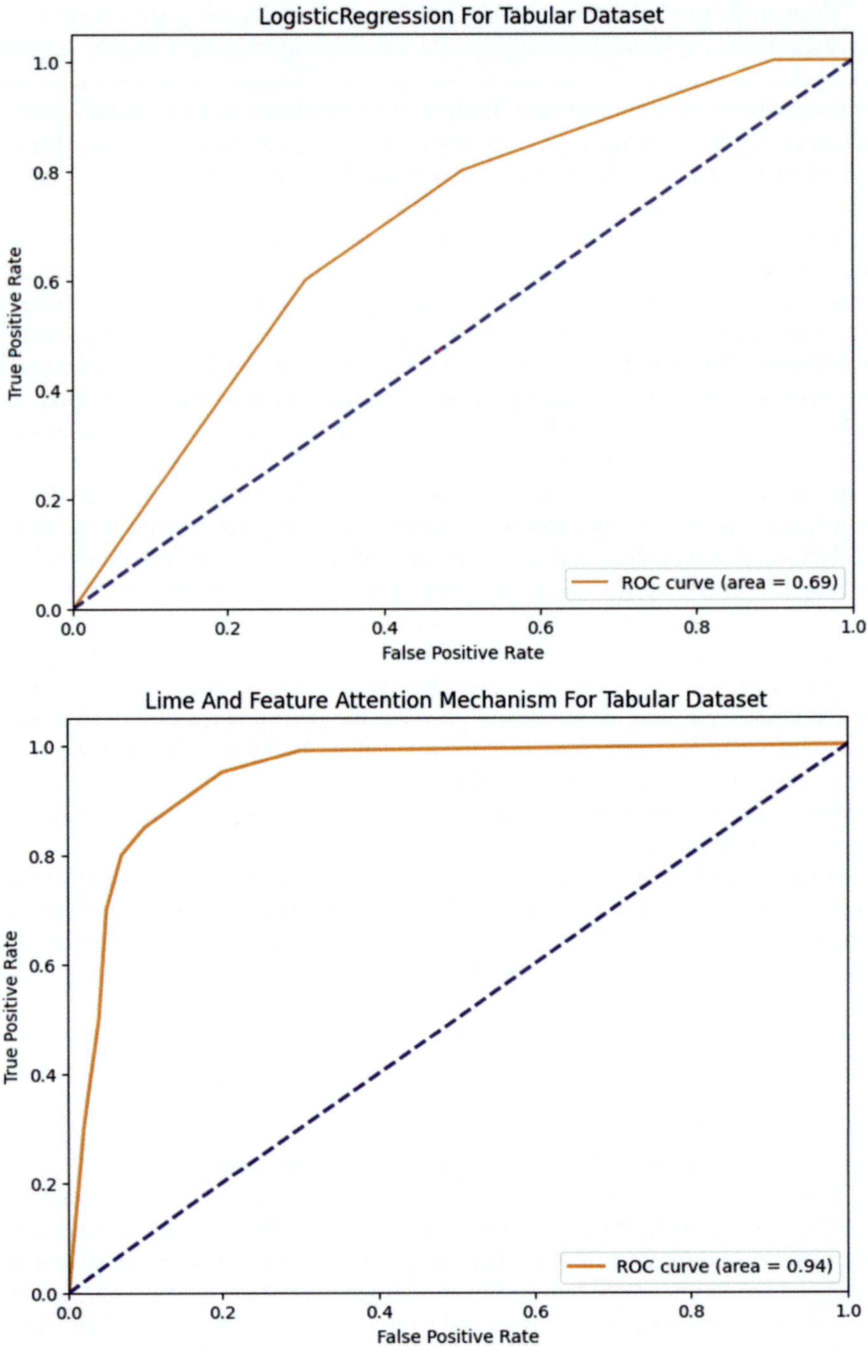

Fig. 9 ROC curve before and after applying LIME + attention mechanism for tabular dataset

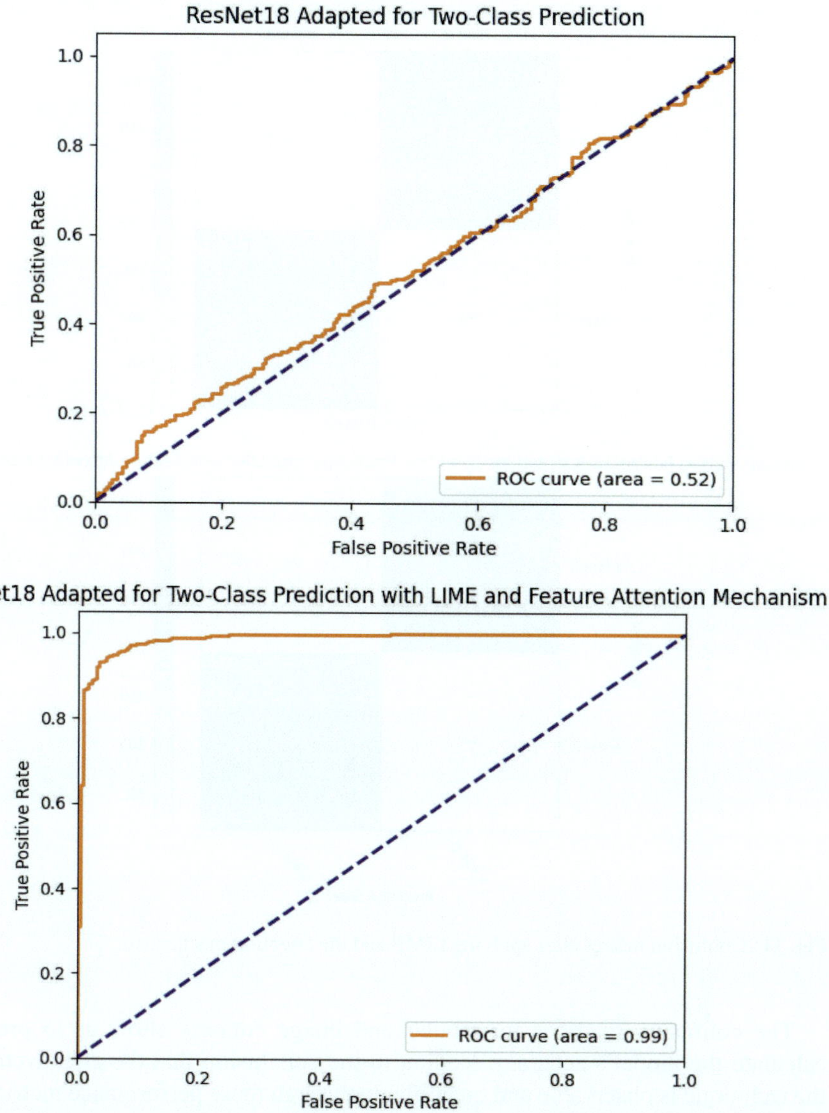

Fig. 10 ROC curve before and after applying LIME + attention mechanism for tabular dataset

selection but also highlight the transformative impact of integrating attention mechanisms into deep learning models, particularly for tailored image classification tasks. This approach underscores the profound potential of targeted model adaptation and the strategic integration of advanced techniques to achieve unparalleled performance in specific classification challenges.

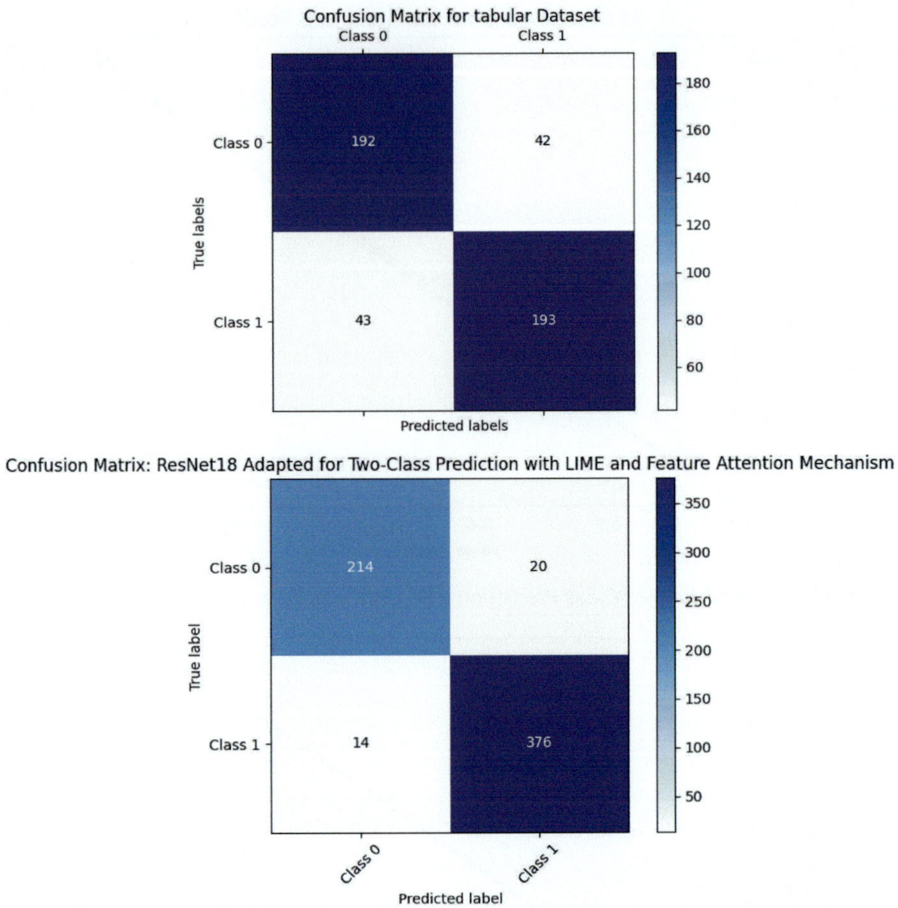

Fig. 11 Confusion matrix after applying LIME and the attention mechanism

The confusion matrices for tabular and image datasets allow us to precisely calculate the model's accuracy, leading to the conclusion that the effectiveness of the technique is observable and quantifiable through these performance metrics (see Fig. 11).

7 Conclusions

The analysis presented above allows us to evaluate the efficacy of our implementation and acknowledge the following outcomes. By extracting the most relevant features from the datasets, we successfully reduced the volume of data used for training our model, focusing solely on pertinent information to predict whether a patient suffers from thoracic issues. By decreasing the number of independent features, we not only reduced the model's training time but also diminished the likelihood of overfitting. The application of the attention mechanism discussed has enabled us to train the model effectively and achieve significantly improved results in both cases. As evidenced by the data, we have managed to increase the accuracy of the model by over 25% in some particular cases. The model's performance is clearly demonstrated in the illustrations of the ROC curves and in the confusion matrices for both cases. Therefore, through this technique, we have trained the model in a more efficient and useful manner, and we have improved the outcome of the clinical data-driven decision support system for thoracic diagnosis.

Declarations

Some journals require declarations to be submitted in a standardized format. Please check the Instructions for authors of the journal to which you are submitting to see if you need to complete this section. If yes, your manuscript must contain the following sections under the heading "Declarations":

- Funding
- Conflict of interest/Competing interests (check journal-specific guidelines for which heading to use)
- Ethics approval and consent to participate
- Consent for publication
- Data availability
- Materials availability
- Code availability
- Author contribution

If any of the sections are not relevant to your manuscript, please include the heading and write "Not applicable" for that section.
Editorial Policies for:
Springer journals and proceedings: https://www.springer.com/gp/editorial-policies
Nature Portfolio journals: https://www.nature.com/nature-research/editorial-policies
Scientific Reports: https://www.nature.com/srep/journal-policies/editorial-policies
BMC journals: https://www.biomedcentral.com/getpublished/editorial-policies

Acknowledgments The authors Darian Onchis and Codruta Istin have been partially supported by the European Union, via the oc1-2024-TES-01-19 sub-grant issued and implemented by the ENFIELD project, under the grant agreement No 101120657.

References

1. Zhang Y, Weng Y, Lund J. Applications of explainable artificial intelligence in diagnosis and surgery. Diagnostics. 2022;12(2):237. https://doi.org/10.3390/diagnostics12020237
2. Huang Q, Yamada M, Tian Y, Singh D, Chang Y. Graphlime: Local interpretable model explanations for graph neural networks. IEEE Trans Knowl Data Eng. 2020;35(7):6968–6972. https://doi.org/10.1109/TKDE.2022.3187455
3. Onchis DM, Costi F, Istin C, Secasan CC, Cozma GV. Method of improving the management of cancer risk groups by coupling a features-attention mechanism to a deep neural network. Appl Sci. 2024;14(1). https://doi.org/10.3390/app14010447
4. Ribeiro MT, Singh S, Guestrin C. Why should I trust you?: Explaining the predictions of any classifier. 2016. arXiv preprint arXiv:1602.04938.
5. Gruber S, Kopper P, Molnar C. Chapter 12: Introduction to local interpretable model-agnostic explanations (LIME). Limitations of interpretable machine learning methods. 2024. https://interaccao2008.xdi.uevora.pt/fc/zugzwang/raw/b6e04759c75c94886c84d0d108ec4edb23349c09/biblio/sota/Limitations%20of%20Interpretable%20Machine%20Learning%20Methods%20%7C%202019.pdf
6. Molnar C. 9.2 Local surrogate (LIME). Interpretable machine learning. 2024. p. 142–153. https://christophm.github.io/interpretable-ml-book/
7. Tanner G. Local model interpretation: An introduction. Model interpretation. 2018. https://gilberttanner.com/blog/local-model-interpretation-an-introduction/
8. Costi F, Onchis D, Hogea E, Istin C. Predictive modeling for diabetes using graphlime. J Med Inform Decis Mak. 2024;30(3):205–16.
9. Bronstein MM, Bruna J, Cohen T, Velič P. A comprehensive guide to graph neural networks. IEEE Signal Process Mag. 2020;37(6):93–112.
10. Lubicz M, Pawelczyk K, Rzechonek A, Kolodziej J. Thoracic surgery data. Donated to the UCI machine learning repository. 2014. https://datasets.aim-ahead.net/dataset/p/UCI_DS_277
11. Siddhartha M. Thoracic surgery dataset. 2017. Available on Kaggle.
12. Chest X-ray Images (Pneumonia). Curated collection of chest radiograph images for automated diagnostic tools development, available on Kaggle.
13. LIME: How to interpret machine learning models with Python. Available at: https://betterdatascience.com/
14. The application of lime in healthcare: Enhancing model transparency and trust. J AI Healthc. 2024.
15. Kim Y, Park H. Enhancing image classification and explainability with object isolation and background randomization. In: Barolli L, editor. Advances on P2P, parallel, grid, cloud and internet computing (3PGCIC 2023). Lecture notes on data engineering and communications technologies. Cham: Springer; 2024. p. 69–80: 189. https://doi.org/10.1007/978-3-031-46970-1_7. https://link.springer.com/chapter/10.1007/978-3-031-46970-1_7
16. Rani LG. Using LIME and tree SHAP to explain decision trees: A case study in explainable AI. Int J Innovative Res Multidiscip Field. 2025:15. https://doi.org/10.2015/IJIRMF/202507012. https://www.ijirmf.com/using-lime-and-tree-shap-to-explain-decision-trees-a-case-study-in-explainable-ai/
17. Enhanced model performance with lime and attention mechanisms across data types. J Mach Learn Innov. 2024.

Explainable Artificial Intelligence for Parkinson's Disease

Tommaso Ruga, Luciano Caroprese, Eugenio Vocaturo, and Ester Zumpano

Contents

Abstract Parkinson's disease (PD) is a complicated neurological condition that calls for a precise diagnosis as well as practical treatment plans. The present state of explainable artificial intelligence (XAI) treatments for Parkinson's disease (PD) is examined in this literature review. In order to find the key aspects, different XAI approaches have been examined. Those approaches are generally used to improve the interpretability and transparency of AI models for Parkinson's disease diagnosis and progression forecasting. Important research is analyzed to show the benefits, drawbacks, and clinical suitability of various XAI techniques. The

T. Ruga (✉) · E. Zumpano
DIMES, University of Calabria, Rende, Italy
e-mail: tommaso.ruga@dimes.unical.it; e.zumpano@dimes.unical.it

L. Caroprese
InGeo, University G. D'Annunzio, Chieti-Pescara, Italy
e-mail: luciano.caroprese@unich.it

E. Vocaturo
CNR-NANOTEC National Research Council, Rende, Italy
e-mail: e.vocaturo@dimes.unical.it

R. Ortale et al. (eds.), *Explainable Machine Intelligence in Healthcare*,
https://doi.org/10.1007/978-3-031-91379-2_8

analysis emphasizes how crucial explainability is to building physician confidence and making it easier to incorporate AI tools into clinical practice. Additionally, the gaps in the existing research are discussed and future directions are proposed.

Keywords Explainable artificial intelligence · XAI · Parkinson's disease · Literature review

1 Introduction

Parkinson's disease (PD) is a rapidly growing public health concern globally, being the second most common neurodegenerative disorder after Alzheimer's disease. Over the past few decades, the prevalence and burden of Parkinson's disease have surged dramatically. In 2019, it was estimated that over 8.5 million individuals were living with PD worldwide, representing a doubling in prevalence over the past 25 years. The disease is associated with both motor symptoms, such as tremors and rigidity, and a wide array of non-motor complications, including cognitive impairment and mental health disorders [1, 2]. The global burden of Parkinson's disease, in terms of years lived with disability (YLDs), has increased significantly. From 1990 to 2019, the age-standardized rates of incidence, prevalence, and YLDs of PD showed substantial upward trends. Specifically, the prevalence of PD has grown at an annual percentage change (EAPC) of 0.52%, with notable increases observed in countries like the United States and Norway [2]. This rise is primarily attributed to the aging population, as the incidence of PD is significantly higher in individuals over the age of 65, and it increases further in those aged over 80 [2]. The impact of Parkinson's disease is profound not only on patients but also on healthcare systems and society at large. In 2019, PD accounted for approximately 5.8 million disability-adjusted life years (DALYs), marking an 81% increase since 2000. Additionally, the number of deaths due to PD has more than doubled over the same period, reaching 329,000 globally in 2019 [1]. These statistics underscore the urgent need for improved management and treatment strategies, especially in light of the predicted continued growth in the disease's burden in the coming decades [3]. Parkinson's disease presents substantial challenges, particularly due to its progressive nature and the complexity of its symptoms, which require comprehensive care and significant healthcare resources. As the global population continues to age, addressing the rising prevalence and burden of PD through effective public health strategies and advancements in medical research becomes increasingly critical. In recent years, due to the increasing demand and the necessity to analyze large amounts of data quickly, artificial intelligence (AI) has emerged as a valuable decision-support tool for domain experts by providing timely diagnoses. However, these experts have shown a certain level of skepticism toward some solutions currently proposed in the literature, mainly because of the overly inexplicable nature of the results obtained. In this context, explainable artificial intelligence (XAI) is positioned as a useful field to enhance the interpretability of these results. XAI techniques, in fact, increase the explainability of not only solutions that use machine learning techniques but also those that use deep learning techniques, which are inherently more unpredictable. This literature review will analyze the main solutions in the field of Parkinson's disease currently present in the literature that make use of XAI techniques. The following work in any case does not set out to be a comprehensive systematic literature review, although it does follow a rigorous selection scheme, but aims to analyze the main solutions currently found in the literature, which refer to the state of the art.

The structure of the work is as follows: After explaining the methodology used for selecting the analyzed studies, a section is presented describing the individual works, with a particular focus not only on the techniques used but also on the datasets utilized. Subsequently, the research results are discussed, focusing on the main XAI techniques used in this field and the types of input data predominantly employed. Finally, the critical issues in the field are highlighted, and possible future solutions are discussed.

The aim of the work is to provide a comprehensive overview of the current state of the art regarding explainable solutions in the context of Parkinson's disease.

2 Methodology

The selection process of the papers analyzed in this review was done following strict steps, in order to rigorously answer the research question proposed below:

- **RQ:** *What are the applications of artificial intelligence for the diagnosis and prevention of Parkinson's disease currently in the state of the art using XAI?*

The process began with searches across multiple academic databases, including PubMed, Scopus, Google Scholar, and ScienceDirect, formalizing the research question **RQ** in a search string as reported in Table 1.

The publication range considered starts from 2020 until April 2024, while in terms of the type of work considered, only peer-reviewed journal articles, conference papers, and significant reports from reputable institutions were considered. The selected studies needed to address the application of AI and machine learning techniques to Parkinson's disease with a specific emphasis on explainability and interpretability. Additionally, only articles available in English were included. Also review articles, editorials, or commentaries without original research data were excluded. The initial search yielded a large number of articles, but downstream of

Table 1 Search string used in databases

Research question	Search string
RQ	*(XAI OR (explainable artificial intelligence) OR (explainable AI)) AND ((parkinson) OR (parkinson's disease))*

the selection process only ten works were chosen for this paper. We first screened the titles and abstracts to eliminate clearly irrelevant studies. This initial screening was followed by a full-text review of the remaining articles to ensure they met the inclusion criteria. For the selected articles, we extracted key information, including the type of AI methods used, the explainability techniques employed, the datasets involved, and the outcomes or findings related to Parkinson's disease diagnosis and treatment. All papers that did not have XAI solutions as their main focus or did not even use them at all were excluded. In a first step, only the titles and abstracts were analyzed to exclude all papers that did not correctly meet the chosen criteria, while in a second step, we went into detail by analyzing the proposed solutions. The third and final stage, which then led to the selection of the ten papers, simply focused on the exclusion of nonpublic papers. An initial analysis of the selected works is proposed in Fig. 1, focusing on the chosen keywords.

By observing the graph, it is not possible to make strong statements. The only evident occurrences, as one might easily think, are those of the keywords "parkinson's disease" and "explainable artificial intelligence (XAI)." Other noteworthy occurrences are those related to the keywords "machine learning" and "convolutional neural network," whose numbers differ by only one occurrence. Therefore, it was not possible to determine at this stage whether the works made more use of machine learning or deep learning techniques. This aspect, along with the XAI techniques used, will be further explored in the final section about the discussion on the results obtained.

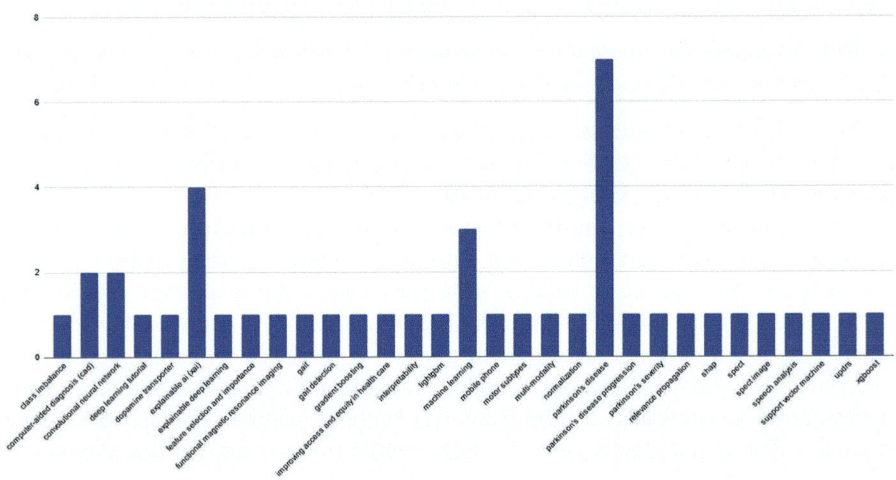

Fig. 1 Keywords distribution in analyzed works

3 Background

3.1 SHapley Additive exPlanations (SHAP)

Shapley Additive exPlanations (SHAP) is a method that makes use of Shapley values from coalitional game theory to explain the prediction of an instance x, which is defined to determine the impact of each feature on the prediction [4]. One of the key features of SHAP is its model-agnostic nature. It can explain the output $f(x)$ of every single machine learning model, including black-box models such as neural networks and ensemble methods, as well as more interpretable models like decision trees and linear regression. SHAP technique can be formalized as shown in Eq. 1:

$$g(z') = \Phi_0 + \sum_{j=1}^{M} \Phi_j z'_j \tag{1}$$

g represents the explanation model, $z' \in M$ denotes the simplified feature, M is the maximum coalition size, and $\varphi_j \in \mathbb{R}$ represents the feature attribution for each individual feature j. In the context of simplified features, an entry of 1 indicates that the corresponding feature value is "present," while an entry of 0 signifies the absence of that feature. A key advantage of SHAP over another technique, i.e., LIME, is that SHAP can provide both local and global explanations, whereas LIME is limited to offering only local explanations. Using a plot of SHAP values, such as summary plots, individual feature importance plots, or dependence plots, explainability can improve. These visualizations help to understand how each feature contributes to the model's predictions and how their values impact the output. SHAP is used to explain the estimations of any AI technique by calculating the contributions of features to the modeling process [5, 6]. SHAP is the result of a combination of different techniques such as Local Interpretable Model-agnostic Explanations, SHAPely sampling values, DeepLift, and QII.

3.2 Local Interpretable Model-Agnostic Explanations (LIME)

Locally Interpretable Model-agnostic Explanations (LIME) is a post hoc explanation technique designed to make any black-box machine learning model more interpretable. LIME works by approximating the complex model with a simpler, interpretable model locally around each prediction. This allows for an understanding of the factors influencing individual predictions, making it possible to explain the behavior of the machine learning model on a case-by-case basis [7]. The importance of features is captured and explained by linear functions as shown in Eq. 2:

$$\text{explanation}(x) = L(f, g, \pi_x) + \Omega(g) \tag{2}$$

The explanation model for the specific instance x is described through the model g, for example, a linear regression model, which minimizes the value of the loss function. Loss L is used to measure of how close the explanation of model g is to the prediction value of the original model f, in this case a ML classifier, whereas the model complexity (g) is kept low by selecting only a few features. The family of available explanations, represented as G, includes options such as all possible linear regression models. The proximity measure π_x defines the extent of the neighborhood around a given instance x that is considered when generating the explanation [8].

LIME allows for the interpretation of any black-box machine learning model for individual predictions. Input data is processed through the black-box model to produce outputs; then, generated data is weighted based on their distance to the target instance. An alternative method, such as linear regression, is then fitted to this weighted dataset, adjusting the sample weights [7].

3.3 Partial Dependence Plot (PDP)

The partial dependence plot (PDP) is a global and model-agnostic explainable AI (XAI) technique. This technique provides an overall explanation of the entire dataset by interpreting the impact of one or more features on the target variable. PDP reveals the marginal effect or contribution of individual features to the predictive value of a black-box model. Unlike global methods, local methods explain the impact of features at the level of local observations. Model-agnostic methods like PDP can be applied to any algorithm or model, guarantying a higher level of flexibility in understanding feature contributions across different types of models. The partial dependence function is defined as shown in Eq. 3:

$$\hat{f}_S(x_S) = E_{X_C}\left[\hat{f}(x_S, X_C)\right] = \int \hat{f}(x_S, X_C)d\mathbb{P}(X_C) \tag{3}$$

The given partial function in the above formula is approximated by calculating averages over the training data as shown in Eq.4:

$$\hat{f}_S(x_S) = \frac{1}{n}\sum_{i=1}^{n} \hat{f}(x_S, x_C^{(i)}) \tag{4}$$

In this context, S represents the set of features of interest–those whose impact on the target variable we aim to understand. Conversely, C is the set containing all other features that are not included in S [9]. PDP is used to examine and interpret the effects of these independent variables on the model's output. This method is used in machine learning solutions as presented in [10].

3.4 Layer-Wise Relevance Propagation (LRP)

Layer-wise relevance propagation (LRP) is an explanation technique applicable to models structured as neural networks [11]. LRP functions by propagating the prediction $f(x)$ backward through the neural network, employing specifically crafted local propagation rules. The propagation process employed by LRP adheres to a conservation principle, ensuring that the information received by a neuron is evenly redistributed to the neurons in the preceding layer. Let j and k be neurons at two consecutive layers of the neural network. Propagating relevance scores $(R_k)_k$ at a given layer onto neurons of the lower layer is done following Eq. 5:

$$R_j = \sum_k \frac{z_{jk}}{\sum_j z_{jk}} R_k \tag{5}$$

The value z_{jk} quantifies the contribution of neuron j to the relevance of neuron k. The denominator ensures the conservation property is maintained during this process. The propagation continues until it reaches the input features. By applying this rule to all neurons in the network, we ensure that the sum of relevance scores for neurons in each layer is equal, i.e., $\sum_j R_j = \sum_k R_k$, maintaining layer-wise conservation. This also upholds the global conservation property, ensuring that $\sum_i R_i = f(x)$.

3.5 Analysis of Variance (ANOVA)

ANOVA, or analysis of variance, is a statistical method used to determine if there are significant differences between the means of three or more independent groups. This method facilitates the identification of at least one group mean that deviates from the others without the necessity of conducting multiple pairwise comparisons [12]. It is based on some key concept, here briefly introduced: independence (the samples must be independent), normality (the data in each group should be approximately normally distributed), and homogeneity of variances (the variances among the groups should be approximately equal). Other key components are the independent variables, called *factors*, and the hypothesis. Hypothesis can be distinguished in two types: null hypothesis (H0), which assumes that all group means are equal, and the alternative hypothesis (H1), which posits that at least one group mean is different. The test statistic for ANOVA is performed calculating *F-statistic*, which is a ratio of the variance between group means to the variance within the groups, and *p-value*. A low *p-value* (typically less than 0.05) indicates that the null hypothesis can be rejected, suggesting significant differences among group means. The *F-statistic* coefficient can be calculated following formula expressed in Eq. 6:

$$F = \frac{MSB}{MSW} \tag{6}$$

MSB stands for the mean square between groups, which is the variance between the group means (between-group variability), and *MSW* stands for the mean square within groups, which is the variance within the groups (within-group variability). There are different types of ANOVA such as *one-way* ANOVA, which compares means across one factor with multiple levels, and *two-way* ANOVA, which examines the influence of two different factors simultaneously.

4 Analyzed Works

4.1 Dataset

The analysis of the datasets used within the work highlighted the critical issues typical of the medical domain when developing artificial intelligence solutions. The sensitive nature of the data and the need to guarantee a high level of privacy for patients always influences the availability aspect. The works almost always use private datasets, and it is very difficult to find valid public datasets for model testing. Table 2 shows the public datasets used by the reviewed works. As can be seen, many works used the dataset, highlighting its validity. This initial analysis shows that many works focus on image analysis, rather than analysis of audio spectra or parametric data. For further details, a more extensive description of the types of data covered in the works is offered in the section on discussion and analysis results.

Table 2 Public datasets used in analyzed works

Ref	Name	Paper	Data description
[13]	Physionet	[16]	Healthy and idiopathic Parkinson's vital data
[14]	PPMI	[19, 23, 25]	Multimodal Data containing DaTSCAN SPECT Parkinson's patients images and vital parameters
[15]	Parkinson Dataset with Replicated Acoustic Features	[24]	Voice recordings of 80 individuals

4.2 Summary of Analyzed Solutions

Khera and Kumar [16] presents a hybrid model for Parkinson's disease (PD) severity evaluation. The work utilizes gait, a biomarker, assessed through vertical ground reaction force (VGRF) data from 72 healthy individuals and 93 Parkinson's patients, from Physionet dataset. Feature importance and partial dependence plot (PDP) analyses elucidate the relevance of gait features, providing valuable insights for clinical applications. A multivariate normalization approach is employed to identify gait differences between PD and non-PD subjects. Normalized gait parameters facilitate comparison across individuals with diverse physical properties, enhancing the evaluation of PD severity. The proposed hybrid model uses a two-step ML workflow to produce results: The first stage is used to distinguish a PD individual from non-PD through a decision tree classifier; the second thereby assesses their severity through ensemble regressors. Proposed approach achieves high accuracy in PD detection (99.39% and 99.9%) and severity assessment (97% and 98.7% coefficient of determination) using leave-one-out cross-validation (CV) and tenfold CV, respectively.

Nazari et al. [17] aimed to address the black-box nature of deep convolutional neural networks (CNN) used in automatic classification of dopamine transporter (DAT) single-photon emission computed tomography (SPECT) images, particularly in patients with uncertain parkinsonian syndromes. CNN achieved high accuracy equal to 95.8%, using 1296 clinical DAT-SPECT images with binary interpretation (normal or reduced) by domain experts. 1008 DAT-SPECT images were used for the training phase, and the remaining 288 were used for the test phase. The method tested layer-wise relevance propagation (LRP) to explain CNN-based classification decisions, proving its effectiveness in this area. In fact, its quick computation time (3 seconds) makes it compatible with busy clinical workflows and particularly indicated in the medical field.

Rahman et al. [18] proposes a web-based framework to enable global Parkinson's disease screening using short speech tasks. Data from 726 participants (PD, 262; non-PD, 464) from diverse locations were collected. Participants spoke a standard phrase, "the quick brown fox jumps over the lazy dog." Standard acoustic features and deep learning-based embeddings were extracted from the speech data. Various machine learning algorithms were trained, and model interpretation techniques, such as Shapley additive explanations, were employed to understand feature importance. The XGBoost model achieved an AUC equal to 0.753, for detecting self-reported PD using standard acoustic features. Analysis revealed that widely used mel-frequency cepstral coefficient features and dysphonia features significantly influenced the model's decision.

Pianpanit et al. [19] discusses the importance of interpretability in deep learning models for medical image analysis, specifically focusing on Parkinson's disease (PD) recognition using single-photon emission computed tomography (SPECT) images. The study uses 2723 SPECT images from the Parkinson's Progression Markers Initiative (PPMI) database, with 1359 images from PD patients and

1364 from normal controls. Deep convolutional neural networks (DCNN) were employed for classification tasks, with specific architectures like Deep PD Net with batch normalization showing the highest accuracy equal to 96.87. The paper explores various interpretation methods for deep learning models, such as guided backpropagation and SHAP, to visualize and interpret the decision-making process of the models. Guided backpropagation outperformed other methods showing a higher mean DICE coefficient.

Pang et al. [20] presents an automatic classifier to distinguish subtypes of Parkinson's disease (PD) using multilevel indices derived from resting-state functional magnetic resonance imaging (rs-fMRI). The study included 96 PD patients, divided into postural instability and gait difficulty (PIGD) subtype and tremor-dominant (TD) subtype. Feature selection methods including two-sample t-test, least absolute shrinkage and selection operator (LASSO), and Spearman's rank correlation coefficient were applied. ML technique used is a support vector machine (SVM), based on both separate and multilevel indices. Feature importance was evaluated using SHAP values. The multilevel rs-fMRI indices based model scores an AUC equal to 0.917 in the validation dataset. Models based on separate indices yielded AUCs ranging from 0.713 to 0.792 in the validation dataset. SHAP analysis identified functional activity and connectivity in the frontal lobe and cerebellum as important features for distinguishing PD subtypes.

Nazari et al. [21] proposes a XAI approach to identify extrastriatal brain regions contributing to the interpretation of dopamine transporter SPECT with 123I-FP-CIT in parkinsonian syndromes. A total of 1306 123I-FP-CIT-SPECT images were retrospectively included, with binary classification as "reduced" or "normal" striatal 123I-FP-CIT uptake by an experienced reader as the standard-of-truth. A custom-made three-dimensional convolutional neural network (CNN) was trained for classification using three different settings: "full image," "striatum only," and "without striatum." CNN's classification performance was tested on 300 SPECT images. Layer-wise relevance propagation (LRP) was employed for voxelwise quantification of relevance in the CNN-based classification. CNN achieved an accuracy score equal to 97.0%, 95.7%, and 69.3% in the "full image," "striatum-only," and "without striatum" settings, respectively. LRP-based relevance maps revealed significant contributions beyond the striatal signal in brain regions including the insula, amygdala, ventromedial prefrontal cortex, thalamus, anterior temporal cortex, superior frontal lobe, and pons.

Ma et al. [22] proposes a gait detection system for Parkinson's disease (PD) patients to aid in diagnosis using an explainable learning architecture. Authors used data from IoT pressure plate, which use sensors to detect the posture of patients, allowing the characteristics of healthy patients to be distinguished from unhealthy ones. The 22 sensoristic features are extracted and divided into 3 categories: force domain, peak domain, and abnormality domain. In order to solve the problem of imbalanced data, SMOTE technique is used in the work. Architecture proposed is based both on machine learning and deep learning techniques, and uses data selection; feature evaluation, such as analysis of variance (ANOVA); and data balancing mechanism, such as SMOTE, for gait detection in PD patients. The solution proposed shows the effectiveness of the implemented workflow reaching an accuracy score equal to 97.32% and 98.41%, with XGBoost and CNN, respectively.

Magesh et al. [23] introduces a machine learning model designed to classify DaTSCAN images as indicative of Parkinson's disease (PD) or not, with a focus on maintaining interpretability. The work uses Parkinson's Progression Markers Initiative (PPMI) dataset, preprocessed through attenuation correction procedures, and a convolutional neural network (CNN) based on VGG16 architecture, through transfer learning technique. The model's predictions are supported by visual explanations generated using Local Interpretable Model-agnostic Explainer (LIME) techniques, which highlight relevant features in the DaTSCAN images. In fact, The LIME technique emphasized the healthy putamen and caudate regions of a non-PD patient as the influential regions in classifying the data as a healthy control. The proposed model achieved an accuracy equal to 95.2% and an AUC equal to 0.94.

Ghaheri et al. [24] presents an ensemble method to detect PD, based on voice signals. Authors used the *Parkinson Dataset with Replicated Acoustic Features* to perform the experiments, which contains 3 repetitions of a 5-second-long phonation made by 80 patients, 40 healthy and 40 with PD, respectively. In order to train the singular models, only high correlated features were selected using Irvine-Pearson Correlation Coefficients. The selected features were used by four machine learning models to perform classification: Extreme Gradient Boosting (XGBoost), Light Gradient Boosting Machine (LightGBM), Gradient Boosting, and Bagging. The final ensemble model was made using hard voting technique. Authors used SHAP technique to score features on the basis of their importance in the diagnosis/classification steps. The solution achieved an F1-score equal to 84.94%.

Junaid et al. [25] introduces a machine learning pipeline to predict the progression of Parkinson's disease (PD) using the Parkinson's Progression Markers Initiative (PPMI) dataset. The dataset includes five time-series modalities, patient characteristics, biosamples, medication history, motor function, and non-motor function data, each with six visits per patient. Statistical features from six visits were calculated for each modality, and various feature selection methods were used to identify the most informative features. Multiple ML models were trained, SVM, RF, ETC, LGBM, and SGD respectively. In order to rigorously detect PD, authors also used data-balancing techniques and an optimization step, a Bayesian optimizer. The XAI technique used in the work is different: SHAP technique was used for global and instance-based explanations, while LIME and SHAPASH were used as local explainers. Performance analysis showed that in the three-class prediction, LGBM model achieved the highest accuracy of 90.73% with non-motor function data, while in the four-class prediction, RF model performed best with a 94.57% accuracy using the same modality. When combining non-motor and motor function data, the LGBM model outperformed others in both experiments with accuracies of 94.89% and 93.73% respectively.

5 Results, Discussion, and Future Perspective

In this section, the XAI solutions for Parkinson's disease analyzed will be discussed. Table 3 provides a brief summary of the main features of the works, with a particular focus on the methodologies used, model development and explainable techniques employed, the performance obtained, and the types of data used.

Analyzing the selected papers, it can be observed that the distribution between the techniques used for the models is rather balanced, with many papers using machine learning techniques and many using deep learning techniques. Little explored is the hybrid domain, where these techniques are combined to create more complex classifiers, as shown in [26]. In contrast, the distribution for XAI techniques is more skewed in favor of the SHAP technique, which is the most widely used, as shown in Fig. 2.

As for the types of data used in the works, most of the works provide solutions that work with images, as shown in Fig. 3. More precisely, many works use single-photo emission computed tomography (SPECT) images, as described in the previous section on individual works. Few works focus on audio data, despite the fact that the authors of [24] demonstrate with their results that it is possible to obtain rigorous results and provide a diagnosis that does not involve the use of imaging techniques or more invasive tests. In particular, this factor, given the nature of the pathology addressed, should not be underestimated and highlights the necessity to investigate the use of techniques that utilize audio data.

Table 3 Analyzed works

Ref	Year	Model	Xai Method	Performances	Input data
[16]	2022	DecisionTree and Ensemble Regressor	PDP	98-99% Accuracy	Vital Parameter/Sensoristic
[17]	2022	CNN	LRP	95.8% Accuracy	Images
[18]	2021	XGBoost and others	SHAP	0.75 AUC	Audio
[19]	2021	DCNN	SHAP	96.87% Accuracy	Images
[20]	2021	SVM	SHAP	0.79-0.91 AUC	Images
[21]	2021	CNN	LRP	97%, 95.7% and 69.3% Accuracy	Images
[22]	2023	XGBoost and CNN	ANOVA	97.32% and 98.41% Accuracy	Vital Parameter/Sensoristic
[23]	2020	VGG16	LIME	95.2% Accuracy	Images
[24]	2023	Ensemble of Gradient Boosting and Bagging based models	SHAP	84.94% F1-Score	Audio
[25]	2023	LightGBM and others	SHAP and LIME	94% Accuracy	Vital Parameter/Sensoristic

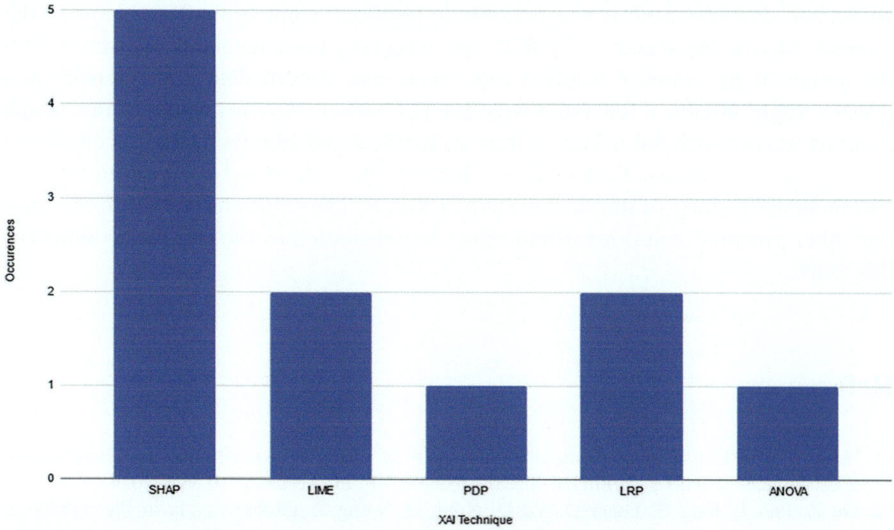

Fig. 2 XAI techniques distribution in analyzed works

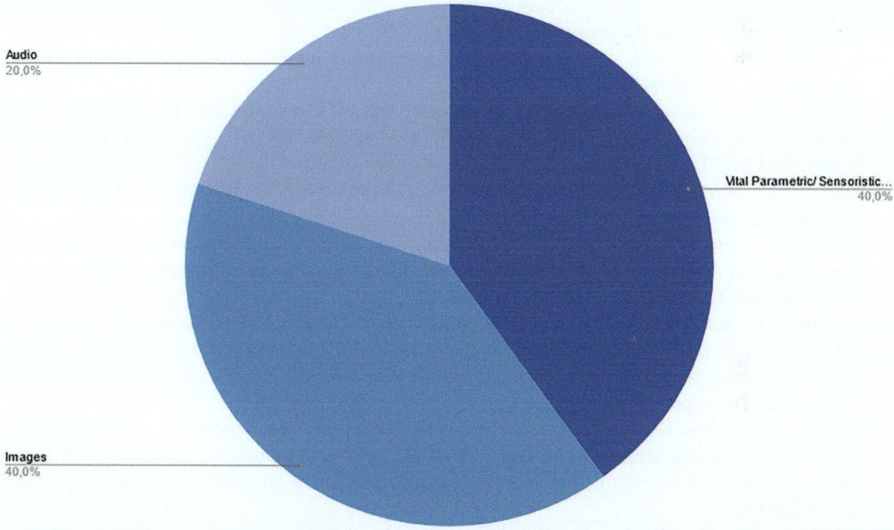

Fig. 3 Input data-type distribution in analyzed works

From the analysis conducted, it is evident that despite the various solutions proposed in the field, much more can still be done. In particular, the final phase of the analysis highlighted the presence of gray areas in the research that could be exploited to propose less invasive solutions using techniques that are still underexplored (such as hybrid solutions). Additionally, from the analysis of the works and datasets used, it was possible to highlight some typical problems of the domain, such as the scarcity of public and especially heterogeneous datasets. Given the nature of the issue, a solution that could ensure both data heterogeneity and privacy might involve a federated structure [27], where data is not stored in a single point on the network but is kept within the medical and care facilities that choose to participate. The proposed work should therefore be understood as a preliminary and comprehensive study of the current state of the art. The solutions just discussed, and any other potential solutions, should thus be considered as the natural evolution of this work.

References

1. "Launch of WHO's Parkinson disease technical brief", https://www.who.int/news/item/14-06-2022-launch-of-who-s-parkinson-disease-technical-brief. Accessed 10 May 2024
2. Ou Z, Pan J, Tang S, Duan D, Yu D, Nong H, Wang Z. Global trends in the incidence, prevalence, and years lived with disability of Parkinson's disease in 204 countries/territories from 1990 to 2019. Front Public Health. 2021;9:776847.
3. "Parkinson's Disease: Challenges, Progress, and Promise", https://www.ninds.nih.gov/current-research/focus-disorders/parkinsons-disease-research/parkinsons-disease-challenges-progress-and-promise. Accessed 11 May 2024.
4. Lundberg SM, Lee SI. A unified approach to interpreting model predictions. Adv Neural Inf Process Syst. 2017;30:4768–77.
5. Mangalathu S, Hwang SH, Jeon JS. Failure mode and effects analysis of RC members based on machine-learning-based SHapley Additive exPlanations (SHAP) approach. Eng Struct. 2020;219:110927.
6. García MV, Aznarte JL. Shapley additive explanations for NO2 forecasting. Ecol Inform. 2020;56:101039.
7. Ribeiro MT, Singh S, Guestrin C. "Why should i trust you?" explaining the predictions of any classifier. In: Proceedings of the 22nd ACM SIGKDD international conference on knowledge discovery and data mining. 2016. pp. 1135–44.
8. Främling K, Westberg M, Jullum M, Madhikermi M, Malhi A. Comparison of contextual importance and utility with lime and Shapley values. In: International workshop on explainable, transparent autonomous agents and multi-agent systems. Cham: Springer International Publishing; 2021, pp. 39–54.
9. Biecek P, Chlebus M, Gajda J, Gosiewska A, Kozak A, Ogonowski D, ... Wojewnik P. Enabling machine learning algorithms for credit scoring–explainable artificial intelligence (XAI) methods for clear understanding complex predictive models. 2021. arXiv preprint arXiv:2104.06735.
10. Friedman JH. Greedy function approximation: A gradient boosting machine. Ann Stat. 2001;29(5):1189–1232.
11. Bach S, Binder A, Montavon G, Klauschen F, Müller KR, Samek W. On pixel-wise explanations for non-linear classifier decisions by layer-wise relevance propagation. PloS One. 2015;10(7):e0130140.
12. Fisher RA. Statistical methods for research workers, 6th ed. 1936.
13. Goldberger AL, Amaral LA, Glass L, Hausdorff JM, Ivanov PC, Mark RG, ... Stanley HE. PhysioBank, PhysioToolkit, and PhysioNet: Components of a new research resource for complex physiologic signals. Circulation. 2000;101(23):e215–e220.
14. Parkinson's Progression Markers Initiative (PPMI). https://www.ppmi-info.org/. Accessed 24 May 2024.

15. Prez C. Parkinson dataset with replicated acoustic features. UCI Mach Learn Repos. 2019. https://doi.org/10.24432/C5701F.
16. Khera P, Kumar N. Novel machine learning-based hybrid strategy for severity assessment of Parkinson's disorders. Med Biol Eng Comput. 2022;60(3):811–28.
17. Nazari M, Kluge A, Apostolova I, Klutmann S, Kimiaei S, Schroeder M, Buchert R. Explainable AI to improve acceptance of convolutional neural networks for automatic classification of dopamine transporter SPECT in the diagnosis of clinically uncertain parkinsonian syndromes. Eur J Nucl Med Mol Imaging. 2022;49:1176–86.
18. Rahman W, Lee S, Islam MS, Antony VN, Ratnu H, Ali MR, ... Hoque E. Detecting parkinson disease using a web-based speech task: Observational study. J Med Internet Res. 2021;23(10):e26305.
19. Pianpanit T, Lolak S, Sawangjai P, Sudhawiyangkul T, Wilaiprasitporn T. Parkinson's disease recognition using SPECT image and interpretable AI: A tutorial. IEEE Sens J. 2021;21(20):22304–16.
20. Pang H, Yu Z, Yu H, Cao J, Li Y, Guo M, ... Fan G. Use of machine learning method on automatic classification of motor subtype of Parkinson's disease based on multilevel indices of rs-fMRI. Parkinsonism Relat Disord. 2021:90:65–72.
21. Nazari M, Kluge A, Apostolova I, Klutmann S, Kimiaei S, Schroeder M, Buchert R. Data-driven identification of diagnostically useful extrastriatal signal in dopamine transporter SPECT using explainable AI. Sci Rep. 2021;11(1):22932.
22. Ma YW, Chen JL, Chen YJ, Lai YH. Explainable deep learning architecture for early diagnosis of Parkinson's disease. Soft Comput. 2023;27(5):2729–38.
23. Magesh PR, Myloth RD, Tom RJ. An explainable machine learning model for early detection of Parkinson's disease using LIME on DaTSCAN imagery. Comput Biol Med. 2020:126:104041.
24. Ghaheri P, Nasiri H, Shateri A, Homafar A. Diagnosis of parkinson's disease based on voice signals using SHAP and hard voting ensemble method. Comput Methods Biomech Biomed Eng. 2024;27(13):1858–74.
25. Junaid M, Ali S, Eid F, El-Sappagh S, Abuhmed T. Explainable machine learning models based on multimodal time-series data for the early detection of Parkinson's disease. Comput Methods Programs Biomed. 2023; 234:107495.
26. Ruga T, Musacchio G, Maurmo D. An ensemble architecture for melanoma classification. Stud Health Technol Inform. 2024;314:183–4.
27. Caroprese L, Ruga T, Vocaturo E, Zumpano E. Revealing brain tumor with federated learning. In: 2023 IEEE international conference on bioinformatics and biomedicine (BIBM). IEEE; 2023, December. pp. 3868–73.

Part III
Case Studies and Applications

Interpreting Convolutional Neural Networks for Brain Tumors: A Transparent Box Approach

Dieine Estela Bernieri Schiavon, Willian de Vargas, Viviane Rodrigues Botelho, Thatiane Alves Pianoschi, and Carla Diniz Lopes Becker

Contents

Abstract Brain tumors present a medical challenge, necessitating precise diagnosis and effective treatment strategies. Early detection is paramount for enhancing patients' quality of life afflicted with brain tumors. Magnetic resonance imaging (MRI) is a powerful diagnostic modality, while convolutional neural networks (CNN) offer adept deep learning algorithms for medical image analysis. However, the complexity and opacity inherent in neural network models make understanding by humans difficult due to the use of hidden layers and the identification of intricate patterns. In this chapter, we employ explainable artificial intelligence (XAI) techniques, specifically saliency maps, to explore the workings of a multiclass CNN model for brain tumor classification. The model was trained on MRI data sourced from three widely utilized datasets, achieving an accuracy of 99% for pituitary tumors, 98% for glioma, and 95% for meningioma. By furnishing transparent and interpretable insights into the behavior of artificial intelligence models, these techniques foster increased transparency and accountability, which is particularly

---

D. E. B. Schiavon (✉) · W. de Vargas · V. R. Botelho · T. A. Pianoschi · C. D. L. Becker
Federal University of Health Sciences of Porto Alegre, Porto Alegre, RS, Brazil
e-mail: dieineb@ufcspa.edu.br; vivianerb@ufcspa.edu.br; thatiane@ufcspa.edu.br; carladiniz@ufcspa.edu.br

R. Ortale et al. (eds.), *Explainable Machine Intelligence in Healthcare*,
https://doi.org/10.1007/978-3-031-91379-2_9

critical in healthcare domains. Given the profound implications and associated risks of artificial intelligence models' decisions on people's lives, it is essential to understand the behavior of convolutional networks, mainly how they arrive at their predictions.

Keywords Artificial intelligence · Brain tumors · Deep learning · Interpretability · Saliency maps · XAI technique

1 Introduction

Understanding the reasons for predictions from deep learning models is an important task, especially in healthcare, as it directly impacts human well-being. Currently, there is a growing demand for explainability in models. The ability to interpret model predictions increases confidence and promotes the responsible and ethical adoption of new technological advances in medicine and healthcare [1]. Techniques that provide transparency when answering the question "How does the model work?" [2] also contribute to interpretability when addressing the question "What can the model say." Lipton [2] distinguished three types of transparency in 2017:

1. Simulability, at the level of the entire model, is when the computational operations of the model are simulatable by a human being in a reasonable time.
2. Decomposability occurs when each part of the model (inputs, parameters, and calculations) admits an intuitive explanation at the level of individual components.
3. Algorithmic transparency at the level of the training algorithm.

In other words, a human can reproduce (simulability) the computing process with a complete understanding of the algorithm (algorithmic transparency), and each part of the model has an intuitive explanation (decomposability). Simulation limits the size and complexity of calculations, decomposition limits the level of abstraction, and algorithmic transparency is not a property of opaque machine learning models, especially artificial neural networks (ANNs) [3].

Explainable artificial intelligence (XAI), used in machine learning applications, is an approach that aims to achieve this level of interpretability. It seeks to create transparent and interpretable models that can provide understandable explanations for decisions or predictions. XAI aims to improve the reliability of artificial intelligence (AI) systems and facilitate collaboration between humans and machines. It also aims to help us create a verifiable science of AI. These techniques include methods for visualizing model internals, feature importance analysis, and rule extraction, among other methods.

This chapter focuses on the saliency maps technique. These techniques can help increase the transparency of AI systems, providing precise and interpretable explanations of their behavior. We used an interpretability technique in a CNN trained on the brain tumor MRI dataset [4]. Tumors of the central nervous system (CNS) result from the abnormal growth of cells in the tissues of these locations [5]. Brain tumors represent 85–90% of all primary CNS tumors [6]. Early cancer detection is a strategy to find the tumor early, thus providing a greater chance of treatment.

2 Saliency Maps

Saliency maps are also known as the vanilla gradient method, pixel attribution maps, and attribution maps. It was introduced by Simonyan, Vedaldi, and Zisserman in 2014 [7]. It provides a straightforward approach to identifying critical areas in an image that a CNN focuses on when recognizing a specific object or class. These maps highlight which parts of the image influence the network's decision-making process for that particular class by examining the gradient within each component of the input relative to the target class. The input features can be input pixels, tabular data, or words [8].

Fundamental work [7] on saliency maps approximates the neural network function as a first-order expansion of a Taylor series, represented by Eq. 1. Given an image I , the CNN assigns it a score $Sc(I)$ for class c . Here, w denotes the derivative of the score for the target class concerning each pixel of the input image "I," while b is the bias term. The derivation of w involves standard input processing followed by backpropagation. Unlike typical backpropagation, which aims to minimize classification errors during training, saliency calculation tracks the output pixel corresponding to the target class.

$$S_c(I) \approx w^T I + b \tag{1}$$

Saliency maps are often generated by techniques such as class activation mapping (CAM) [9], Gradient-weighted class activation mapping (Grad-CAM) [10], and local interpretable model-agnostic explanations (LIME) [11]. Our preliminary study [12] utilized feature visualization, CAM, and Grad-CAM techniques with heatmaps to interpret a binary model for brain tumor classification. In our subsequent study [1], we employed only LIME for the interpretability of a multiclass model aimed at identifying gliomas, meningiomas, and pituitary tumors.

In addition, there are two approaches for generating saliency maps: integrated gradients [13] and SmoothGrad [14]. These alternative methods provide complementary perspectives on interpreting model predictions and identifying influential features in input data. They are independent of CNN architecture.

The integrated gradients algorithm [13] is an attribution technique that calculates the contribution of each input feature to the output of a deep neural network model. It calculates the integral along a linear path from the reference input to the current input, efficiently approximating the integral by a sum of gradients at points along that path. Integrated gradients can be visualized to highlight the distinctive characteristics of the input.

SmoothGrad [14] is a technique that aims to improve the stability and interpretability of saliency maps by adding a smoothing effect to the calculated gradients. It performs multiple gradient passes over the perturbed input (added with Gaussian noise) and calculates the average of the gradients obtained in each pass. SmoothGrad suggests visualization results.

Each technique can produce saliency maps, aiding in interpreting decisions made by convolutional neural network models. These insights into how the model processes inputs and generates predictions contribute to our understanding of the model's behavior, thereby enhancing human comprehension. This work will use examples of saliency maps enabled with Grad-CAM and LIME techniques.

3 Applications

CAM and Grad-CAM techniques are commonly used to explain models in computer vision. The CAM technique is limited in that it does not apply to all architectures; only those that use global average pooling can use it. Grad-CAM can be used in any CNN architecture.

The LIME technique is more flexible and can be used in computer vision and tabular data. Similarly, the SmoothGrad technique can also be used in computer vision and Natural Language Processing (NLP).

The integrated gradient is a technique broadly applicable to any differentiable model, such as images, text, or structured data. It has many use cases, including understanding feature importance, identifying data occurrence, and debugging model performance [13].

Examples of computer vision applications include activity recognition, segmentation, object recognition and detection, image captioning, advertising, novice training, surveillance, and patient diagnosis.

For our case study, "we will use a trained model previously presented in our paper [1]. The model was trained on a dataset from a public repository, which is widely used in current brain tumor classification works. The main aspects and results will be presented, focusing on the interpretability of this model's predictions. The model prediction quality is very similar to those of several other published articles [15, 16] and surpasses previous studies [17–19].

4 Dataset

The brain tumor MRI dataset is available in a public repository [4]. It comprises 7023 magnetic resonance imaging (MRI) images of the human brain, divided into two subsets: training (5712 images) and test (1311 images). The images were classified into glioma, meningioma, no tumor, and pituitary. This dataset is composed of results from merging information from three distinct datasets [20–22].

5 Model Description

The CNN used in the experiments is an ensemble model for multiclass classification [1]. The model is composed of four binary classification models. These models were designed to classify glioma x meningioma, glioma x pituitary, meningioma x no tumor, and meningioma x pituitary. In the second phase, an ensemble model combined binary models for multiclass classification. The architecture of each submodel includes convolutional and pooling layers, starting with 32 filters, a 5×5 kernel, and ReLU activation function, followed by a repeated pattern, increasing the filters to 64, 128, and then returning to 64, with max pooling for dimensionality reduction. Global average pooling was applied to reduce the image dimensionality to the global average, facilitating the training of the subsequent dense layer. A dropout layer with a 0.2 rate was used for regularization to prevent overfitting. The final dense layer has 4 units for multiclass classification, using softmax activation function and assigning probabilities to the output classes. The adopted optimizer was Adam, with a learning rate of 0.001, and the loss function is sparse_categorical_crossentropy.

6 Training

The training process was carried out in two phases. The first phase involved the training of binary classification models. To evaluate the performance of the models on different subsets of data, we employ three repeated fivefold cross-validation, except on submodel number 4, where we apply two repeated fivefold cross-validation.

After training the binary models, we created an ensemble model to leverage each binary model's knowledge in multiclass classification, considering the specialized information each model acquired during training. The learning curves highlight the model's performance during the 3 repeated holdouts for 20 training epochs (Fig. 1).

After completing the training and validation phases, the ensemble model underwent an additional 30 epochs of training using all previously employed training and validation images. Subsequently, the model was assessed using a distinct test dataset to evaluate its generalization capability. Images were used to classify brain tumors [23], divided into four categories: glioma, meningioma, no tumor, and pituitary. During the tests, a set of 1103 images was used.

The model's performance is illustrated through the confusion matrix (Fig. 2), which provides the predictions for each class.

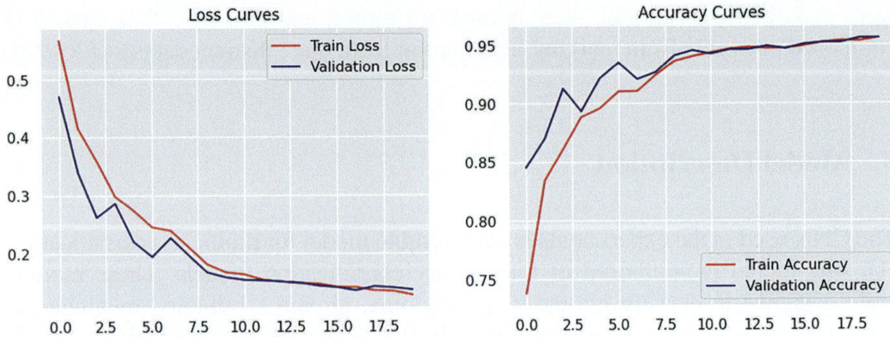

Fig. 1 Learning curves of the multiclass ensemble model [1]

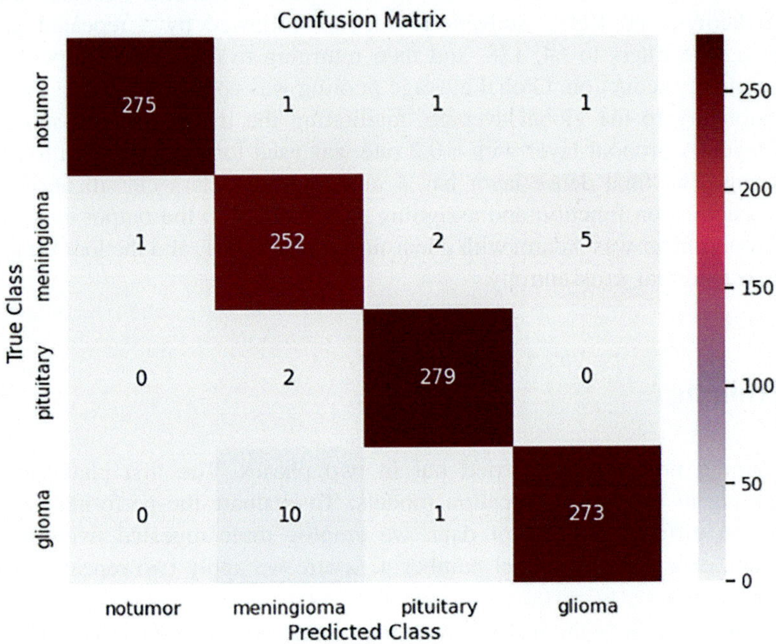

Fig. 2 Model test confusion matrix [1]

7 Model Explainability

We use the saliency maps interpretability methodology to explain the model's final predictions. The use of this technique allows the user to understand how the model makes predictions. The maps highlight the input regions that most influence the model output, enabling a deeper and more transparent understanding of the model's decision-making process. This visualization increases confidence in the model results and makes it easier to identify potential biases or areas for improvement.

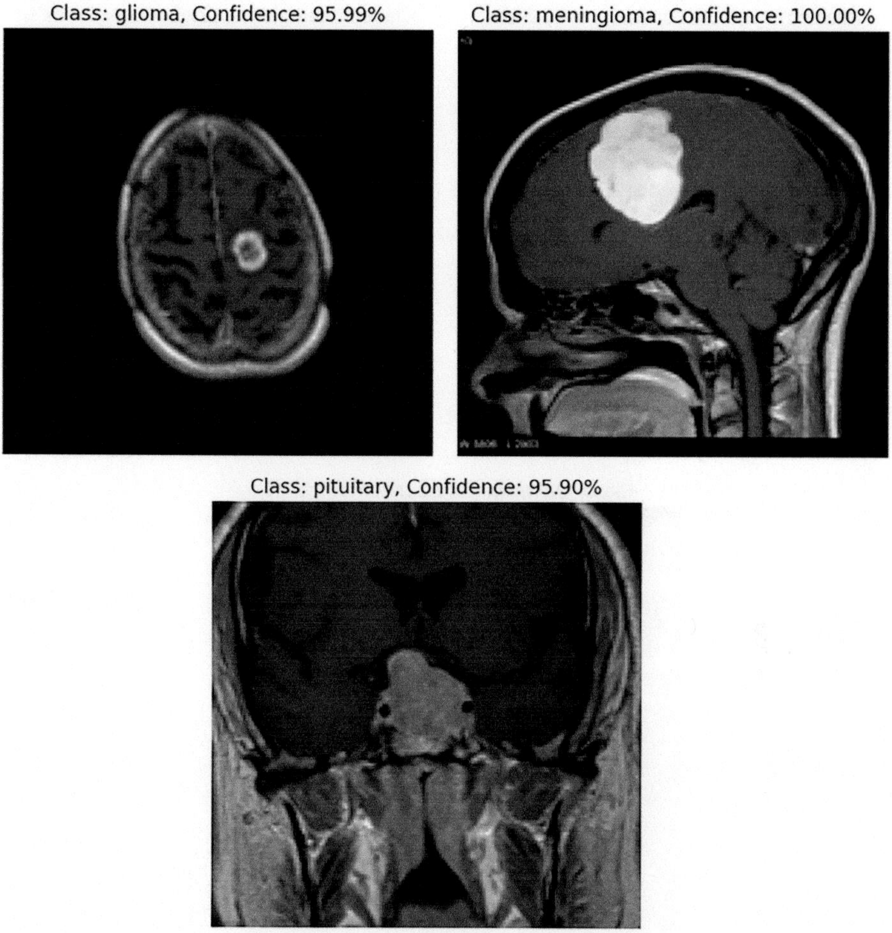

Fig. 3 Example of correct predictions with high confidence

In Fig. 3, we show some correct predictions made by the model used; on the other hand, in Fig. 4, we present some incorrect predictions. In Figs. 5, 6, 8, and 9, we will perform interpretability through saliency maps using the prediction images from Figs. 3 and 4. In Fig. 7, we use other images with model predictions to interpret through saliency maps but with another way to present.

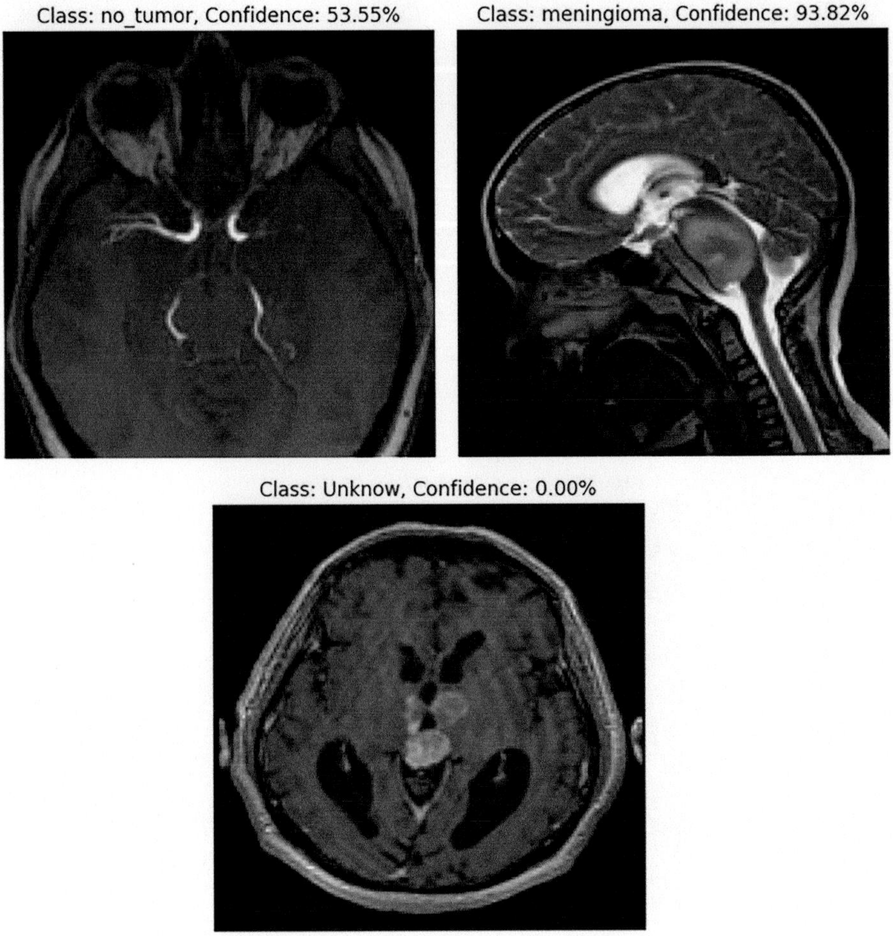

Fig. 4 Example of incorrect predictions—*real class: glioma*

7.1 Saliency Maps with Grad-CAM

We start analyzing predictions by exploring saliency maps with the Grad-Cam technique. It is important to highlight that the images utilized for explainability were sourced from publicly available and untrained repositories, ensuring an impartial evaluation of the ensemble model. The selection of images from health websites [24] aims to assess the model's ability to generalize to novel images, thereby simulating real-world scenarios and ensuring the classification's robustness across diverse contexts outside the known environment during training.

Grad-CAM [10] is an explainable AI technique employed in CNNs to pinpoint the pivotal regions within an image that influenced a specific class prediction.

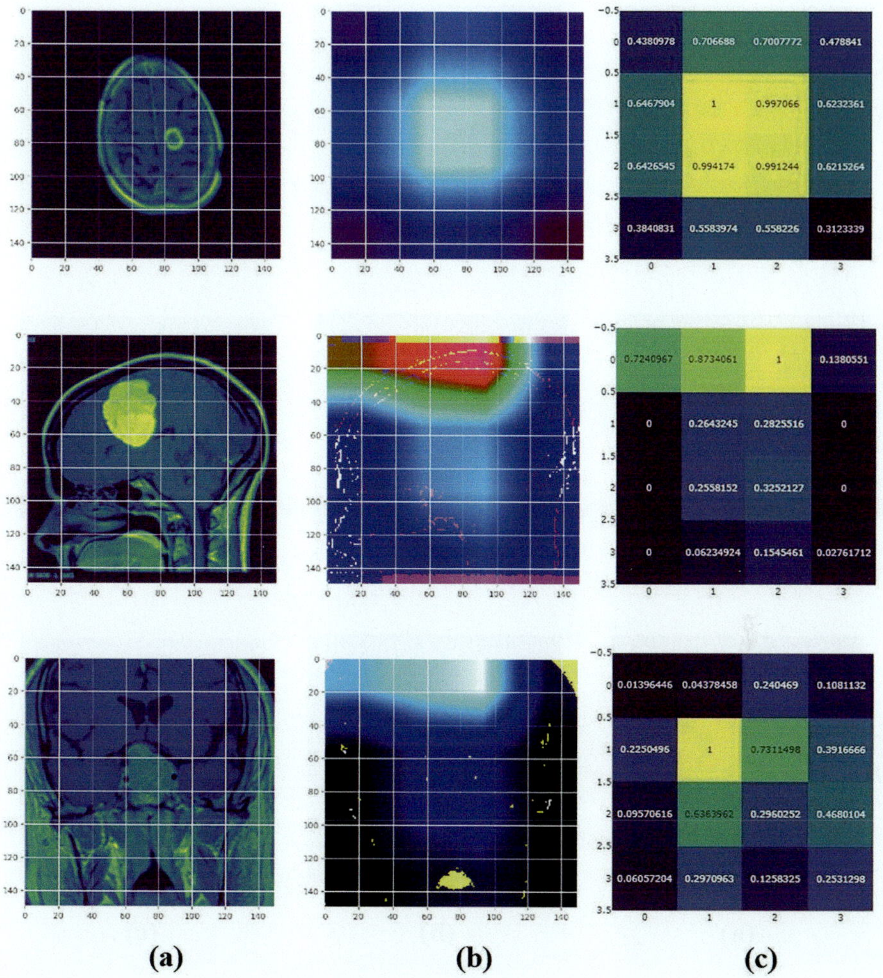

Fig. 5 Saliency maps of correct predictions. (**a**) Original images from the Web. (**b**) The heatmaps are generated by the Grad-CAM technique through a gradient-weighted class activation map. (**c**). Saliency maps with value assignment

By leveraging gradient information from the final convolutional layer of the network, Grad-CAM crafts a heatmap, highlighting these critical areas. Grad-CAM is versatile and can be applied to diverse CNN architectures.

The saliency maps highlight areas of the image that guide the classification provided by CNN. In Figs. 5 and 6, the images on the left (a) are the original images, in the middle (b) are the heat maps generated, and on the right (c) a saliency map, with colors and numbers that represent, on a scale of 0 to 1, where 1 is more significant for classification, and consequently 0 is less significant. The interpretation is that the greater the absolute value of the gradient, the stronger the

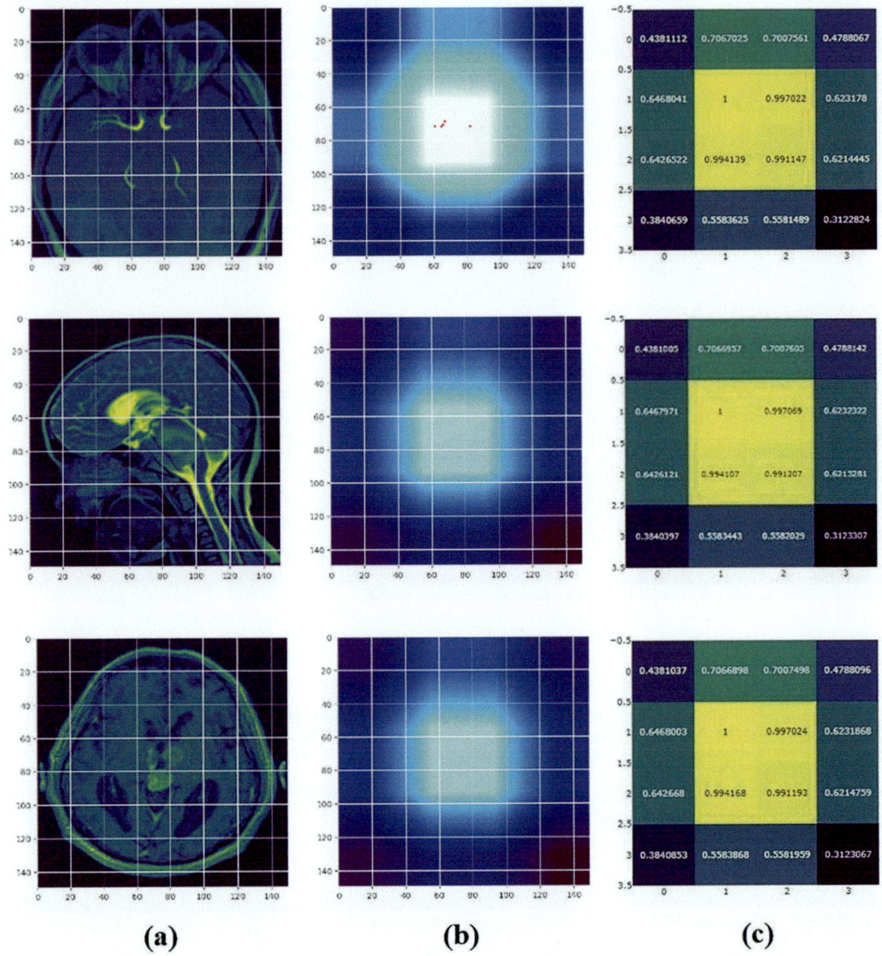

Fig. 6 Saliency maps of incorrect predictions for glioma. (**a**) Original images from the Web. (**b**) The heatmaps are generated by the Grad-CAM technique through a gradient-weighted class. (**c**) Saliency maps with value assignment. Here, unlike correct predictions, where the contribution of pixels is in different parts of the image, incorrect predictions show that the model focused more on the pixels in the center of the images

effect of a change in this pixel. The model paid attention to the final prediction in the areas where the values are 1 or around these.

Figure 7 demonstrates four prediction analyses: two correctly predicted classes, "no tumor" (a) and "glioma" (b), and two incorrect predictions, "pituitary" (c), misclassified as "meningioma" and "meningioma" (d) misclassified as "no tumor." Using this saliency map, we can merge the original image with the map to generate an attention map, highlighting the areas of the image that the model assigns greater importance to its classification [25].

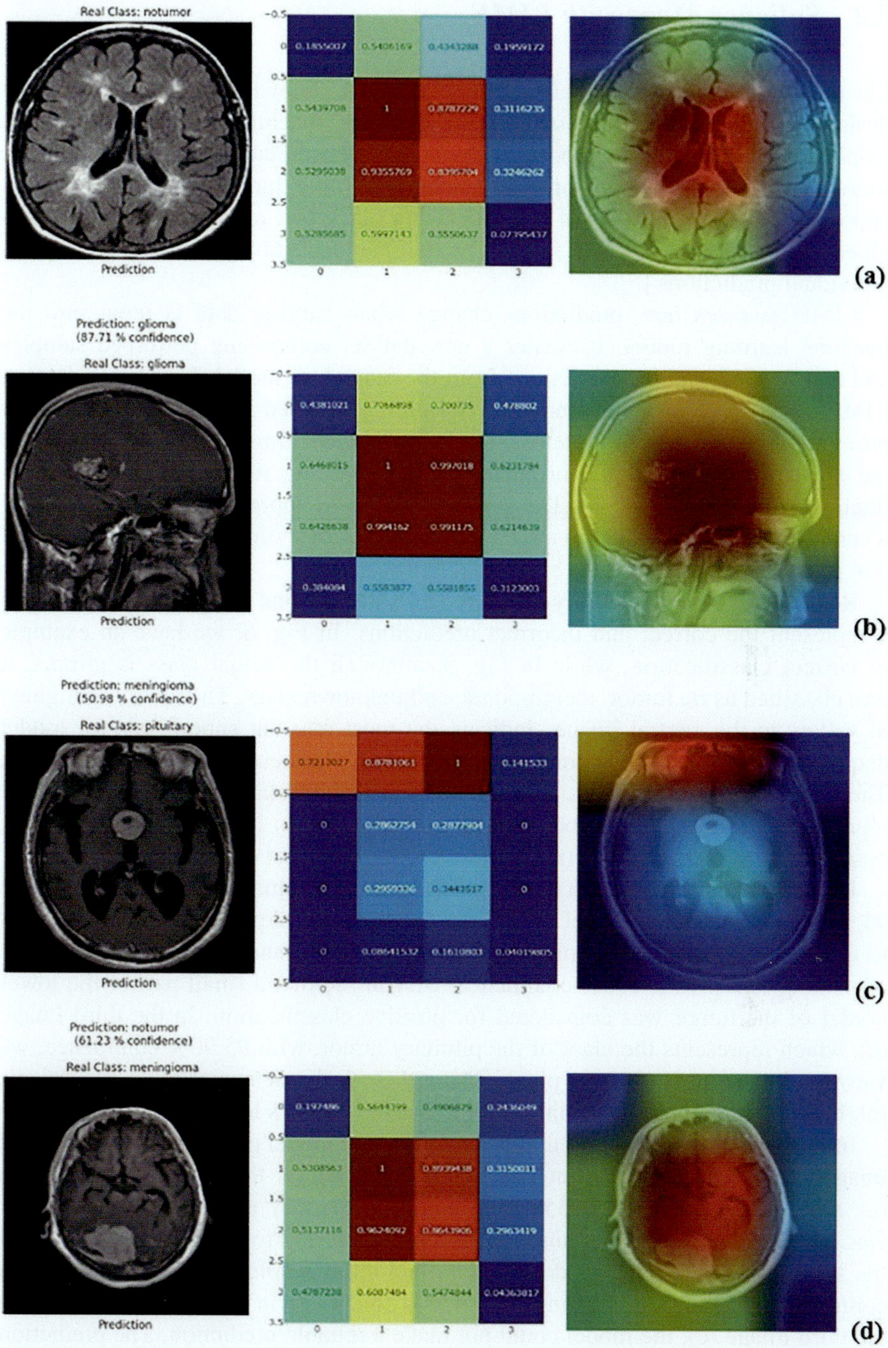

Fig. 7 Attention maps to correct and incorrect model predictions. *Correct classes*: (**a**) no tumor and (**b**) glioma. *Incorrect classes*: (**c**) pituitary to meningioma and (**d**) meningioma to no tumor

7.2 Saliency Maps with LIME

Local interpretable model-agnostic explanations, known as LIME [8], were designed to provide interpretability for complex machine learning models. It employs local surrogate models, which are interpretable models explaining individual predictions from opaque machine learning models. These surrogates approximate the predictions of the underlying black box model. Unlike training a global surrogate model, LIME focuses on training local surrogate models to explain individual predictions [5].

LIME assesses how predictions change when varying data is input into the machine learning model. It creates a new dataset comprising perturbed samples and their corresponding predictions from the black box model. Using this dataset, LIME trains an interpretable model by weighting sampled instances based on their proximity to the instance of interest. The learned model aims to closely approximate the local predictions of the original machine learning model, prioritizing local fidelity over global accuracy. The primary goal is to approximate the behavior of a complex black box model in a localized region with a simpler, transparent model that is easier to interpret.

Regarding the explainability of the model's predictions with LIME, Figs. 8 and 9 represent the correct and incorrect predictions. In Fig. 8, we have an example of correct classification, while in Fig. 9, although the actual class is glioma, it was classified as no tumor, meningioma, and unknown class. The areas highlighted in yellow in the central images indicate the most relevant superpixels for model decision, with these critical areas highlighted while the rest of the image is hidden. The third image, on the right, presents the same interpretation but with a different representation style. Green and red play a crucial role in interpretation, indicating positive (green) and negative (red) contributions to correct classification.

In the first image (a), which represents the class of gliomas in the axial plane, with 95.99% confidence, the model considered the right lateral part of the image, closest to the tumor. In the second image (b), in the sagittal plane, representing the class of meningiomas, with 100% confidence, we can see that a small part of the lower border of the tumor was considered for positive classification. In the third image (c), which represents the class of the pituitary tumor, with 95.90% confidence, we view the image in the coronal plane, where there is the demarcation of superpixels (highlighted in yellow), providing insight into the tumor's location.

In Fig. 9, we used LIME to understand incorrect model predictions. The original images are all of gliomas, but the model misclassified them. In the first image (a), with a confidence of 53.55%, the model incorrectly predicted that no tumor was present, denoting uncertainty in the prediction due to the low confidence. In the second image (b), the model misclassified the example as meningioma with a confidence of 93.82%, indicating the model's conviction in the misclassification. In the third image (c), the model could not make a reliable prediction. The prediction is labeled as "unknown," meaning that the model could not identify any classes with significant certainty, so no confidence is associated with this prediction.

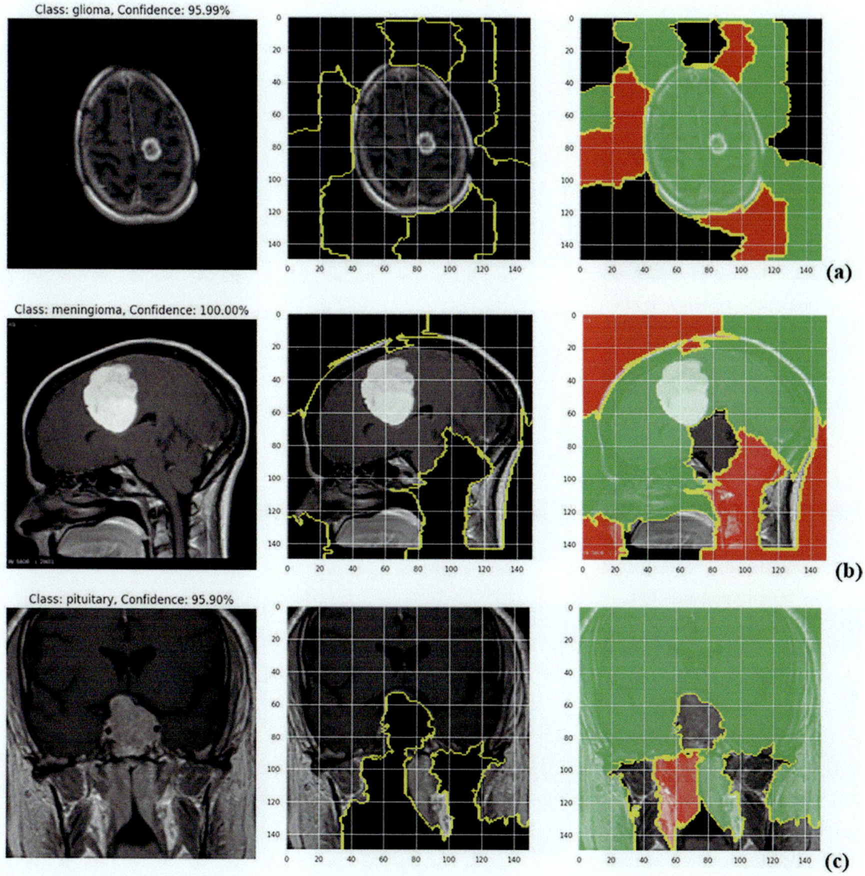

Fig. 8 Saliency maps with LIME and correct predictions: (**a**) glioma classification with 95.99% confidence, (**b**) meningioma classification with 100% confidence, and (**c**) pituitary classification with 90.90% confidence

8 Challenges and Limitations

Exhausting all the techniques used on saliency maps and conducting an extensive review of the literature on saliency maps is beyond the scope of this work. Instead, we focus on presenting the most widely used techniques for leveraging saliency maps in computer vision, adopting a practical approach. It allows us to assess our AI models or other architectures as desired.

Upon completing the analysis, we have compiled a list of critical considerations. Recognizing these constraints can help avoid misinterpretations and maximize the model analysis's potential.

For this study, we used a previously trained simple CNN and applied the techniques to only a few images. Generating and interpreting saliency maps in large

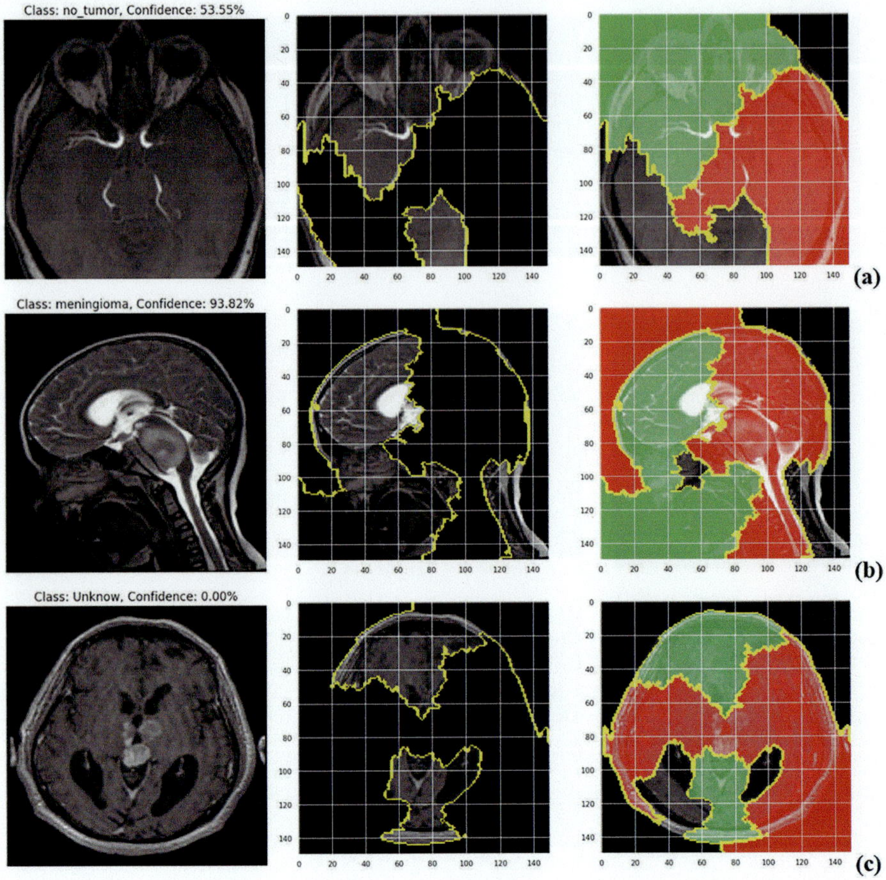

Fig. 9 Saliency maps with LIME and incorrect predictions—*actual class*: glioma: (**a**) no tumor classification with 53.55% confidence, (**b**) meningioma classification with 93.82% confidence, and (**c**) unknown classification with no confidence

datasets or complex models can be computationally intensive and time-consuming, limiting their applicability in large-scale scenarios.

Interpreting the model's mistakes can be complex, especially when a very large area is highlighted on the map (Fig. 6). Even with a visual explanation, the potential for each evaluator's interpretation to differ is a significant factor to consider, highlighting the need for further research and discussion in this area.

The maps highlight regions considered important for the model's prediction but do not necessarily provide a comprehensive understanding of the model's decision-making process. Further in-depth investigations are often necessary to grasp the underlying mechanisms [26].

9 Conclusion

XAI techniques have gained prominence in the scientific community. Beyond providing mathematical metrics such as accuracy, sensitivity, and specificity, additional considerations are needed, especially in healthcare. By applying these techniques, we can better understand what the model is considering; however, this interpretation still depends on the observer's interpretive ability when analyzing the generated images.

Interpretability techniques for computer vision, whether through the visualization of features or saliency maps, contribute to unveiling the opacity inherent in deep learning models, making the model's predictions more transparent to human eyes. They also provide a more accurate understanding of the decision-making process in diagnosing and treating brain tumors.

This chapter has taken a more practical approach, highlighting the importance of understanding the predictions of AI models applied to human health, especially in the context of brain tumor diagnosis. Integrating AI into clinical practice requires the development of accurate models and a human understanding of how these models work and how we can interpret their predictions.

Therefore, continued progress in developing AI models for medical diagnosis and improving healthcare professionals' understanding of how to use these models for science is essential to ensuring that AI supports the diagnosis and treatment of diseases such as brain tumors for the benefit of humans.

References

1. Vargas W, Schiavon DEB, Botelho VR, Pianoschi TA, Becker CDL. Improving automatic classification of brain tumors with deep learning techniques. J Health Inf. 2024;
2. Lipton ZC. The mythos of model interpretability: in machine learning, the concept of interpretability is both important and slippery. Queue. 2018;16(3):31–57.
3. Carabantes M. Black-box artificial intelligence: an epistemological and critical analysis. AI & Soc. 2020;35(2):309–17.
4. Nickparvar M. Brain Tumor MRI Dataset [Data set]. *Kaggle*; 2021.
5. INCA. Central nervous system cancer. National Cancer Institute – INCA; 2022. https://www.gov.br/inca/pt-br/assuntos/cancer/tipos/sistema-nervoso-central
6. National Cancer Institute. Adult central nervous system tumors treatment. National Cancer Institute. Cancer.gov; 2019. https://www.cancer.gov/types/brain/hp/adult-brain-treatment-pdq
7. Simonyan K, Vedaldi A, Zisserman A. Deep inside convolutional networks: visualising image classification models and saliency maps; 2013. arXiv preprint arXiv:1312.6034
8. Molnar C. Interpretable machine learning. Github.io; 2019. https://christophm.github.io/interpretable-ml-book
9. Chollet F. Deep learning with python. Shelter Island: Manning Publications Co.; 2017.
10. Selvaraju RR, Cogswell M, Das A, Vedantam R, Parikh D, Batra D. Grad-cam: visual explanations from deep networks via gradient-based localization. In: Proceedings of the IEEE international conference on computer vision; 2017. p. 618–26.

11. Ribeiro MT, Singh S, Guestrin C. "Why should I trust you?" explaining the predictions of any classifier. In: Proceedings of the 22nd ACM SIGKDD international conference on knowledge discovery and data mining; 2016, August. p. 1135–44.
12. Schiavon DEB, Becker CDL, Botelho VR, Pianoski TA. Interpreting convolutional neural networks for brain tumor classification: an explainable artificial intelligence approach. In: Brazilian conference on intelligent systems. Cham: Springer Nature Switzerland; 2023. p. 77–91.
13. Sundararajan M, Taly A, Yan Q. Axiomatic attribution for deep networks. In: International conference on machine learning. PMLR; 2017. p. 3319–28.
14. Smilkov D, Thorat N, Kim B, Viégas F, Wattenberg M. Smoothgrad: removing noise by adding noise; 2017. arXiv preprint arXiv:1706.03825
15. Rasool M, Ismail NA, Boulila W, Ammar A, Samma H, Yafooz WM, Emara AHM. A hybrid deep learning model for brain tumour classification. Entropy. 2022;24(6):799.
16. Rasool M, Ismail NA, Al-Dhaqm A, Yafooz WM, Alsaeedi A. A novel approach for classifying brain tumours combining a squeezenet model with svm and fine-tuning. Electronics. 2022;12(1):149.
17. Mahajan N, Chavan H. A robust approach for brain tumor detection using transfer learning. In: 2023 5th international conference on inventive research in computing applications (ICIRCA). IEEE; 2023. p. 429–34.
18. Gómez-Guzmán MA, Jiménez-Beristaín L, García-Guerrero EE, López-Bonilla OR, Tamayo-Perez UJ, Esqueda-Elizondo JJ, et al. Classifying brain tumors on magnetic resonance imaging by using convolutional neural networks. Electronics. 2023;12(4):955.
19. Özkaraca O, Bağrıaçık Oİ, Gürüler H, Khan F, Hussain J, Khan J, Laila UE. Multiple brain tumor classification with dense CNN architecture using brain MRI images. Life. 2023;13(2):349.
20. Sartaj B, Ankita K, Prajakta B, Sameer D, Swati K. Brain tumor classification (MRI). *Kaggle*. 2020
21. Cheng J. Brain tumor dataset. *figshare. Dataset, 1512427*(5); 2017.
22. Hamada A. Br35h:: Brain tumor detection 2020. Version 5; 2020.
23. YOLOv5_Brain_Tumor_Detection_And_Classification Dataset. Roboflow Universe; 2023. https://universe.roboflow.com/college-tsy2r/yolov5_brain_tumor_detection_and_classification
24. Radiopaedia. Radiopaedia.org, the wiki-based collaborative Radiology resource. Radiopardia.org; 2019. https://radiopaedia.org/
25. Kluge N. Nkluge-correa/TeenyTinyCastle. GitHub; 2024. http://github.com/Nkluge-correa/TeenyTinyCastle
26. Yang S, Berdine G. Interpretable artificial intelligence (AI)–saliency maps. Southwest Respir Crit Care Chron. 2023;11(48):31–7.

Evaluation of Explainability Methods in Medical Image Analysis

Toygar Tanyel and Ilkay Oksuz

Contents

Abstract In the field of medical image analysis, artificial intelligence (AI) has made significant research-level advancements and is gradually being integrated into real-world applications. Explaining the decisions made by AI in the context of medical image analysis is crucial. However, it is equally important that these explanations are evaluated quantitatively with appropriate metrics to be able to quantify the success of various explainability methods. Considering that many medical decisions are subjective and vary with experience, we can deduce how challenging yet necessary this task is. In this chapter, we present the various

T. Tanyel (✉)
Biomedical Engineering Graduate Program, Istanbul Technical University, Istanbul, Turkey
e-mail: tanyel23@itu.edu.tr

I. Oksuz
Department of Computer Engineering, Istanbul Technical University, Istanbul, Turkey
e-mail: oksuzilkay@itu.edu.tr

R. Ortale et al. (eds.), *Explainable Machine Intelligence in Healthcare*,
https://doi.org/10.1007/978-3-031-91379-2_10

challenges and the multitude of algorithms designed to make this quantitative evaluation meaningful. We explain the current state of the literature for quantitative evaluation metrics in medical image analysis and highlight the limitations with possible future directions.

Keywords Explainable artificial intelligence · Quantitative evaluations · Machine learning · Deep learning · Medical imaging · Medical image analysis

1 Concept

In today's world, although artificial intelligence provides significant practical benefits in many fields [1–3], it is still far from replacing doctors in the field of medical imaging—even when integrated into hospitals [4–8]. One of the primary reasons for this can be exemplified as follows: a radiologist can take responsibility for a wrong decision and manage the process; but when artificial intelligence makes a wrong decision, who will take responsibility for it? Furthermore, when artificial intelligence works alongside doctors, it is crucial that it does not mislead them and conveys its benefits in a manner compatible with human nature [9]. Can we say why the machine made a particular decision? If we can, how can we measure whether our way of explaining is rational and truly reflects what the model considers important? At this point, various algorithms and guidelines capable of making these measurements to a certain extent come into play [10, 11]. Although the algorithms and methods presented here are far from being an exhaustive list, we will focus on the quantitative and qualitative measurement methods frequently used in the literature.

2 Introduction

This chapter focuses on methods that allow us to "measure" which current explanation methods are superior, why, and in what contexts. This enables us to present our model's decisions to doctors in the most effective way for various medical tasks, including medical image analysis, disease classification, tissue segmentation, and many other tasks [12–14].

We introduce evaluation methods from different perspectives, beginning with quantitative metrics (Sect. 4): fidelity, consistency, robustness, faithfulness, and localization will be briefly explained. We focus on evaluating the most commonly used saliency-based explanation methods for medical imaging decisions using two useful localization metrics. We proceed to discuss popular qualitative evaluation metrics (Sect. 5) where quantitative measurement is not feasible, including expert reviews, user studies, focus groups, and case studies (Fig. 1).

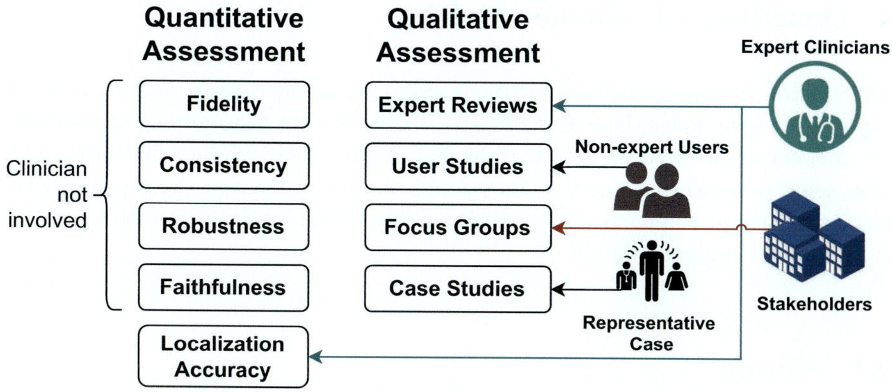

Fig. 1 Covered assessment methods. Both quantitative and qualitative assessment techniques are utilized to assess the performance of the explainability tools in AI for medical imaging analysis

3 Challenges in Evaluating Explainability

Explainability in medical image analysis is a challenging area for computer scientists and radiology experts. In everyday life, usually the sole focus is the decision, and the complexity of the system of AI-based technologies is overlooked. However, in the context of medical imaging—where the data inherently contains a richer bit depth and more information than normal images—the necessity of designing models to focus on the very different characteristics of medical data becomes apparent. Moreover, the "how" part of the decision-making process is the most critical aspect. As the system becomes more complex, it becomes increasingly difficult to accurately reflect and measure this reflection of the decision.

The inherent complexity of medical data, including various additional dimensions (e.g., spatial, time), the need for different requirements for various modalities (e.g., MRI, mammography, CT scans), necessitates a specialized approach in the design of AI models and in the decisions they make, especially if a precise methodology is known, following a specific logical process. Dragging this complexity to a common benchmark for all medical image analysis is also not meaningful due to this complexity. Analyzing decisions and improving models require deep understanding in the medical field and technical knowledge in AI.

Another challenge is subjective assessments. This issue arises from the fact that each doctor has different levels of expertise, different experiences, and different education and skills and that each patient is different from each other. How to translate decisions that contain medical subjectivity to the AI side, and how to evaluate AI decisions, makes the issue even more complex because even if AI makes the correct decision, the individuals interacting with it will still be clinicians with different experiences.

4 Quantitative Evaluation Metrics

This section introduces various metrics used to assess the quality and reliability of explanation techniques. Due to the lack of a general consensus among researchers, we conceptualize these metrics here to demonstrate their fundamental principles; thus, keep in mind that many studies adapt them for their specific purposes. We place a particular emphasis on the quantitatively robust localization metrics, which are discussed in greater detail.

4.1 Fidelity

For the evaluation of explanation fidelity in machine learning models, particularly in terms of how explanations reflect the model's decision-making process, Velmurugan [15] provides a detailed path for understanding fidelity. To generalize this concept, fidelity measures the extent to which a model's explanations accurately reflect its actual outputs. High fidelity indicates that the explanation is a true representation of the model's decision-making process.

4.1.1 Evaluation

The fidelity of an explanation can be evaluated by comparing the model's performance on the original input versus a perturbed version of the input, where the perturbation is informed by the explanation. For example, if an explanation highlights specific features as important, modifying or obscuring these features should notably impact the model's output if the explanation is faithful.

A generalized formula to compute fidelity is as follows:

$$F = \frac{1}{N} \sum_{i=1}^{N} \left| f(x_i) - f(x_i') \right| \tag{1}$$

where:

- N is the number of instances evaluated,
- $f(x)$ is the model's output for the original instance x,
- $f(x')$ is the model's output for the perturbed instance x', and
- $|\cdot|$ denotes the absolute difference, indicating the impact of the explanation-guided perturbation on the model's output.

Example Usage

In the context of medical image analysis, consider a model tasked with classifying X-ray images. The fidelity of an explanation that identifies specific regions as critical for a pneumonia diagnosis can be evaluated by measuring the change in the model's confidence when these regions are masked or altered:

$$F_{\text{example}} = |p - p'| \tag{2}$$

Here, p and p' represent the model's confidence in the pneumonia diagnosis before and after perturbation, respectively. A significant change in confidence indicates high fidelity of the explanation, validating its relevance and accuracy.

4.2 *Consistency*

Consistency in explanation methods ensures that identical inputs produce the same explanations, reflecting the determinism of these methods [16]. This attribute is important, particularly in approaches focusing only on model inputs and outputs without considering the model's internal workings. This principle ensures that the explanations are reliable and can be trusted across similar instances, or even across different models that behave similarly. Honneger [17] discusses these concepts in detail, highlighting the importance of reliable explanatory methods in machine learning.

4.2.1 Evaluation

Consistency can be quantified by comparing explanation similarities, using metrics like cosine similarity and Pearson correlation. For intra-model consistency

$$C_{\text{intra}} = \frac{1}{N}\sum_{i=1}^{N} \text{sim}(E(x_i), E(x_i')) \tag{3}$$

And for inter-model consistency

$$C_{\text{inter}} = \frac{1}{N}\sum_{i=1}^{N} \text{sim}(E_{M_1}(x_i), E_{M_2}(x_i)) \tag{4}$$

where N is the number of instances, $E(x)$ the explanation for instance x and $\text{sim}(\cdot)$ a similarity measure.

Example Usage

An example involves assessing the consistency of explanations by two AI models detecting pulmonary tuberculosis from chest X-rays. High inter-model consistency scores between different model architectures indicate a reliable focus on pertinent regions for diagnosis.

4.3 Robustness

Robustness quantifies the stability of an explanation against small perturbations or variations in the input data [18]. In the context of medical image analysis, robust explanations are crucial, as they ensure that minor changes in input, such as noise or variations in imaging techniques, do not lead to significantly different interpretations.

Robustness in explainable AI aims to measure the resilience of explanations to changes in the input data. This metric is essential for ensuring that explanations remain consistent and reliable, even in the face of data variability common in clinical settings.

4.3.1 Evaluation

To quantitatively assess robustness, one approach involves introducing small, controlled perturbations to the input data and observing the variation in the generated explanations. The smaller the variation, the higher the robustness. This can be mathematically expressed as

$$R = 1 - \frac{1}{N} \sum_{i=1}^{N} \frac{\|E(x_i) - E(x_i + \delta)\|}{\|\delta\|} \quad (5)$$

where:

- N is the number of input instances evaluated,
- $E(x)$ represents the explanation for input x,
- δ is a small perturbation added to the input x_i,
- $\|\cdot\|$ denotes a norm indicating the magnitude of change in the explanation due to δ.

Example Usage

An application of robustness evaluation can be found in models predicting diabetic retinopathy from fundus photographs. By applying slight variations to these photographs (e.g., adjusting brightness or adding noise) and measuring how much the explanations (e.g., saliency maps highlighting areas of interest) change, researchers can quantify the robustness of the explanations provided by the AI model.

4.4 *Faithfulness*

Faithfulness measures the extent to which the explanations or features identified as important by an explainability method truly influence the model's output [19]. In medical image analysis, faithful explanations ensure that the features highlighted as significant for a diagnosis or classification task correspond to those actually used by the model.

The concept of faithfulness is central to the utility and reliability of explainable AI. It assesses whether the explanation accurately reflects the causative reasoning of the model rather than merely being correlated with its predictions.

4.4.1 Evaluation

Quantitative assessment of faithfulness can involve interventions on the input data based on the explanation and observing the impact on the model's output. A commonly used metric is the drop in model accuracy or confidence when features deemed important by the explanation are altered or removed:

$$F = \frac{1}{N} \sum_{i=1}^{N} \left(p(y|x_i) - p(y|x_i') \right) \tag{6}$$

where:

- N is the number of instances,
- $p(y|x)$ is the model's prediction probability for the correct class y given input x,
- x_i' represents the altered input where features identified as important are modified.

Example Usage

An example of evaluating faithfulness in AI models could involve a deep learning system used for detecting malignant tumors in MRI scans. By systematically occluding areas highlighted as important by the explanation method and measuring the subsequent impact on the model's prediction confidence, researchers can assess the faithfulness of the explanations. A significant decrease in confidence when important features are occluded would indicate high faithfulness.

4.5 *Localization Accuracy*

Localization accuracy assesses the precision with which explainability methods highlight regions of interest (ROIs) within medical images, correlating these with actual pathological or clinically relevant features. Among the metrics to evaluate this precision, the Ground Truth Overlap Ratio (m_{gt}) [20] and the Pointing Game [21] are good examples with their direct applicability in medical image analysis.

4.5.1 Ground Truth Overlap Ratio (m_{gt})

m_{gt} is a quantitative metric designed to measure the accuracy with which explainable AI models identify clinically relevant features in medical images. It assesses the degree of spatial agreement between the salient regions highlighted by the model's explanation mechanisms and the actual pathological areas marked by expert annotations.

The implementation of the m_{gt} metric involves generating binary masks from both the model's explanation output—focusing on the top p most salient pixels or regions—and the ground truth annotations for comparison:

$$\text{Ground Truth Overlap Ratio}(m_{gt}) = \frac{\text{Sum of Overlapping Pixels}}{\text{Total Ground Truth Pixels}} \tag{7}$$

! Significance

m_{gt} can serve as an important benchmark for ensuring the reliability of AI-driven diagnostics in healthcare, indicating the model's alignment with medical expertise in pinpointing disease indicators.

Example Usage

Consider a deep learning model developed to detect and localize tumors in mammography images (Fig. 2). The m_{gt} metric can be applied to evaluate how well the model's explanations (e.g., highlighted tumor regions in saliency maps) overlap with tumor boundaries as delineated by radiologists in the ground truth annotations.

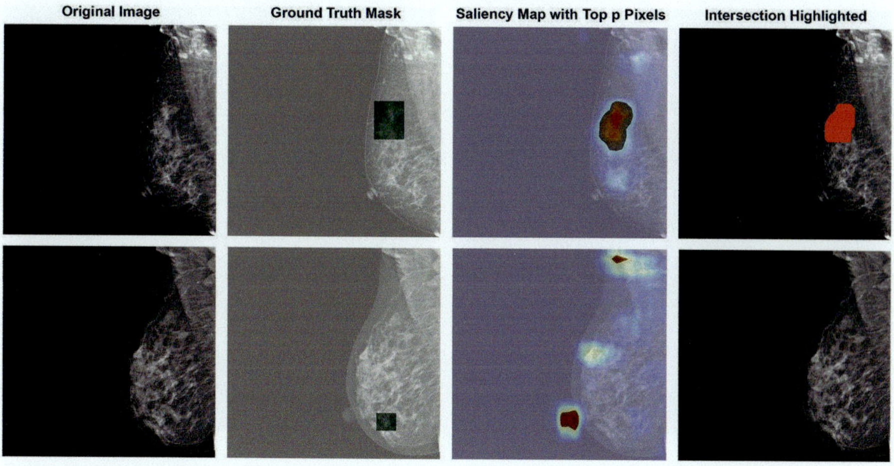

Fig. 2 Ground Truth Overlap on right mediolateral oblique (MLO) mammograms: Two examples showing the top-p overlapping pixels, where p equals the ground truth bounding box area. The first example accurately identifies the tumor area; the second does not

4.5.2 Pointing Game

The Pointing Game is a straightforward yet powerful metric for evaluating the localization accuracy of explainability methods, particularly in highlighting regions of interest (ROIs) that are crucial for the model's decision-making process, which is utilized in general computer vision tasks [22].

The Pointing Game assesses whether the most salient point or region identified by the explainability method coincides with the actual target or pathological feature as defined by ground truth annotations. It simplifies the evaluation to a binary outcome—either a hit or a miss—based on whether the identified point lies within the ground truth region (Fig. 3).

The accuracy of the Pointing Game is quantified as the ratio of hits to the total number of cases (hits and misses):

$$\text{Accuracy} = \frac{\text{Number of Hits}}{\text{Number of Hits} + \text{Number of Misses}} \tag{8}$$

! Significance

The Pointing Game offers an intuitive gauge of whether AI models are zeroing in on the correct features for their diagnoses, critical for clinical applications where precise localization of pathologies is necessary.

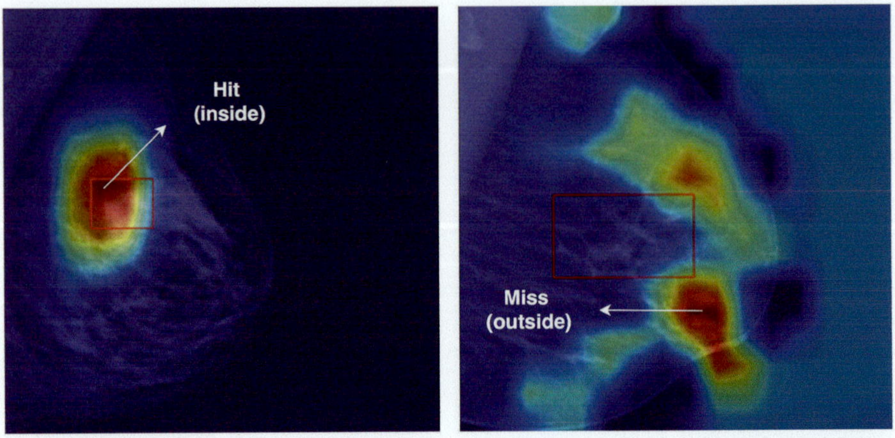

Fig. 3 Hit or miss: Grad-CAM analysis on left MLO mammograms [23]. Left, accurate localization of relevant area; right, localization is off

5 Qualitative Evaluation Methods

Qualitative evaluation methods focus on assessing the subjective aspects of explainability in medical image analysis. These methods involve human interpretation and judgment to evaluate the usability, relevance, and comprehensibility of explanations provided by AI models [10].

5.1 Expert Reviews

Expert reviews are a crucial qualitative method where domain experts such as radiologists or pathologists assess the quality and utility of the explanations generated by AI systems [24]. These reviews help in understanding whether the explanations align with expert knowledge and clinical expectations.

5.1.1 Implementation

During expert reviews, a panel of clinical experts is presented with both the AI-generated explanations and the corresponding medical images. Experts evaluate the explanations based on criteria such as clarity, relevance to the diagnosis, and alignment with medical reasoning.

Example Usage

Consider a scenario where an AI model designed for early detection of glaucoma from optical coherence tomography (OCT) scans undergoes expert review. A group of ophthalmologists evaluates the AI-generated explanations to determine how effectively these explanations map to known pathological features of glaucoma. They specifically assess whether the explanations detail changes in the optic nerve and retinal nerve fiber layer, which are critical for diagnosing the disease. The review focuses on the clarity of these explanations and their utility in supporting early clinical decision-making, ultimately assessing whether the AI's insights contribute to enhanced patient management and trust in automated systems.

5.2 *User Studies*

User studies involve collecting feedback from the end-users of AI systems, such as medical practitioners who may not be experts in AI but use these tools in clinical settings. The focus is on evaluating the explanations' interpretability and the impact they have on the users' decision-making process [10, 25, 26].

5.2.1 Implementation

In user studies, practitioners use the AI system in a controlled environment to perform specific tasks while relying on the provided explanations. Their interaction, decision-making process, and final judgment are monitored and analyzed to gather insights into the practical utility of the explanations.

Example Usage

Consider a user study involving a range of healthcare providers including nurses and general practitioners, using an AI system designed for early detection of diabetic retinopathy in retinal images. Participants, who may not have specialized knowledge in AI, would use the system during routine screenings. The study would focus on how these healthcare providers interpret the AI-generated explanations and the extent to which these explanations affect their diagnostic decisions, particularly in terms of confidence and perceived accuracy.

5.3 Focus Groups

Focus groups gather a diverse set of stakeholders, including clinicians, technicians, and even patients, to discuss and evaluate the explanations from various perspectives. This method is especially valuable for gauging the broader impacts and acceptance of explainability in AI.

5.3.1 Implementation

A moderator leads the focus group, facilitating discussions about the AI explanations based on specific cases or general usage. Participants share their perceptions, potential concerns, and the perceived value of AI explanations in enhancing understanding or trust.

Example Usage

Imagine a focus group session evaluating a new AI system designed to predict the progression of Alzheimer's disease from MRI scans. The group includes neurologists, radiology technicians, and family members of patients. The moderator prompts discussions on how the AI's explanations influence the clinicians' diagnostic strategies, the technicians' workflow, and the families' comprehension of the disease's trajectory. Special attention is given to whether the explanations help in building trust among patients and their families, and if they make the clinical information more accessible to nonspecialists. This session aims to identify gaps in explanation clarity and explore potential improvements in AI communication to support informed decision-making.

5.4 Case Studies

Case studies involve in-depth analysis of specific instances where AI explanations played an important role in medical decision-making. They provide detailed narratives that help illustrate successes and challenges in real-world applications [27].

5.4.1 Implementation

Selecting representative cases where the AI's explanation significantly influenced the clinical outcome, researchers document the entire process, from the initial image analysis to the final treatment decision, highlighting the role of AI explanations.

Example Usage

Consider a case study documenting the use of AI in diagnosing pediatric pneumonia from chest X-rays. This particular study focuses on a challenging case where traditional diagnostic methods provided ambiguous results. The AI system analyzed the X-ray and highlighted subtle patterns not immediately apparent to radiologists. The explanation provided by the AI guided the pediatrician to a correct diagnosis and timely treatment, potentially preventing severe complications. The case study details the decision-making process, the AI's role in enhancing diagnostic accuracy, and how the explanation facilitated a better understanding of the disease presentation, thus emphasizing the critical value of explainable AI in enhancing patient outcomes.

6 Summary and Future Directions

This chapter provides a brief review of the evaluation of explainability methods for AI in medical imaging. The critical importance of explainable AI in healthcare is highlighted due to the potential consequences of decisions based on AI interpretations, especially when these decisions must integrate seamlessly with human judgment.

The complexity of medical data and the subjective nature of medical decision-making present unique challenges in the application of AI. As we continue to integrate AI into medical imaging, reviewing explainability methods uncovers significant opportunities for further research and development. Future work in this field can focus on several key areas to enhance the effectiveness and trustworthiness of AI systems in healthcare setting:

- **Standardization of Metrics:** Develop standardized metrics for universal application across imaging modalities and specialties.
- **Interdisciplinary Collaboration:** Enhance collaboration between AI developers, clinicians, and regulatory bodies to align AI explanations with clinical needs.
- **Diversity and Bias Mitigation:** Focus on ensuring AI systems provide equitable and unbiased explanations across diverse patient groups.
- **Real-time Explanation Methods:** Advance real-time explanatory methods that support swift clinical decision-making.
- **Ethical and Legal Frameworks:** Explore ethical and legal aspects to define accountability clearly in AI-assisted decisions.
- **Longitudinal Studies:** Implement longitudinal studies to evaluate the impact of AI explanations on clinical outcomes and patient satisfaction over time.

By addressing these future directions, researchers and developers can significantly improve the reliability, transparency, and effectiveness of AI in medical imaging, thereby aligning technology advancements with the core goals of patient-centered care.

Acknowledgments This work was supported by the Health Institutes of Türkiye (TUSEB) 2022-EKG-01 Program (Project No: 20101).

References

1. Zhang C, Lu Y. Study on artificial intelligence: The state of the art and future prospects. J Ind Inf Integr. 2021;23:100224.
2. Yin J, Ngiam KY, Teo HH. Role of artificial intelligence applications in real-life clinical practice: Systematic review. J Med Internet Res. 2021;23(4):e25759.
3. Barragán-Montero A, Javaid U, Valdés G, Nguyen D, Desbordes P, Macq B, Willems S, Vandewinckele L, Holmström M, Löfman F, et al. Artificial intelligence and machine learning for medical imaging: A technology review. Phys Med. 2021;83:242–56.
4. Ahuja AS. The impact of artificial intelligence in medicine on the future role of the physician. PeerJ. 2019;7:e7702.
5. Shuaib A, Arian H, Shuaib A. The increasing role of artificial intelligence in health care: Will robots replace doctors in the future? Int J Gen Med. 2020;891–6.
6. Jin W, Li X, Hamarneh G. Evaluating explainable AI on a multi-modal medical imaging task: Can existing algorithms fulfill clinical requirements? In: Proceedings of the AAAI conference on artificial intelligence, vol. 36, Vancouver. 2022. pp. 11945–53.
7. Brady AP, Allen B, Chong J, Kotter E, Kottler N, Mongan J, Oakden-Rayner L, Dos Santos DP, Tang A, Wald C, et al. Developing, purchasing, implementing and monitoring AI tools in radiology: Practical considerations. A multi-society statement from the ACR, CAR, ESR, RANZCR & RSNA. Insights Imaging. 2024;15(1):16.
8. Alis D, Tanyel T, Meltem E, Seker ME, Seker D, Karakaş HM, Karaarslan E, Öksüz İ. Choosing the right artificial intelligence solutions for your radiology department: Key factors to consider. Diagn Interv Radiol. (Ankara, Turkey). 2024.
9. Neri E, Coppola F, Miele V, Bibbolino C, Grassi R. Artificial intelligence: Who is responsible for the diagnosis? La radiologia medica, 2020;125(6):517–521.
10. Jin W, Li X, Fatehi M, Hamarneh G. Guidelines and evaluation of clinical explainable AI in medical image analysis. Med Image Anal. 2023;84:102684.
11. Lekadir K, Feragen A, Fofanah AJ, Frangi AF, Buyx A, Emelie A, Lara A, Porras AR, Chan A-W, Navarro A, et al. Future-AI: International consensus guideline for trustworthy and deployable artificial intelligence in healthcare. arXiv preprint arXiv:2309.12325. 2023.
12. Singh A, Sengupta S, Lakshminarayanan V. Explainable deep learning models in medical image analysis. J Imag, 2020;6(6):52.
13. Najjar R. Redefining radiology: A review of artificial intelligence integration in medical imaging. Diagnostics. 2023;13(17):2760.
14. Wang AQ, Karaman BK, Kim H, Rosenthal J, Saluja R, Young SI, Sabuncu MR. A framework for interpretability in machine learning for medical imaging. IEEE Access, 2024;12:53277–53292.
15. Velmurugan M, Ouyang C, Moreira C, Sindhgatta R. Developing a fidelity evaluation approach for interpretable machine learning. arXiv preprint arXiv:2106.08492. 2021.
16. Nauta M, Trienes J, Pathak S, Nguyen E, Peters M, Schmitt Y, Schlötterer J, Van Keulen M, Seifert C. From anecdotal evidence to quantitative evaluation methods: A systematic review on evaluating explainable AI. ACM Comput Surv. 2023;55(13s):1–42.
17. Honegger M. Shedding light on black box machine learning algorithms: Development of an axiomatic framework to assess the quality of methods that explain individual predictions. arXiv preprint arXiv:1808.05054. 2018.
18. Alvarez Melis D, Jaakkola T. Towards robust interpretability with self-explaining neural networks. Proceedings of the 32nd International Conference on Neural Information Processing Systems. Adv Neural Inf Proces Syst. 2018;31:7786–7795.

19. Wolf TN, Bongratz F, Rickmann A-M, Pölsterl S, Wachinger C. Keep the faith: Faithful explanations in convolutional neural networks for case-based reasoning. In: Proceedings of the AAAI conference on artificial intelligence, vol 38, Vancouver, 2024. pp. 5921–5929.
20. Szczepankiewicz K, Popowicz A, Charkiewicz K, Nałęcz-Charkiewicz K, Szczepankiewicz M, Lasota S, Zawistowski P, Radlak K. Ground truth based comparison of saliency maps algorithms. Sci Rep. 2023;13(1):16887.
21. Ozer C, Oksuz I. Explainable image quality analysis of chest x-rays. In: Medical imaging with deep learning. 2021.
22. Zhang J, Bargal SA, Lin Z, Brandt J, Shen X, Sclaroff S. Top-down neural attention by excitation backprop. Int J Comput Vis. 2018;126(10):1084–1102.
23. Cerekci E, Alis D, Denizoglu N, Camurdan O, Seker ME, Ozer C, Hansu MY, Tanyel T, Oksuz I, Karaarslan E. Quantitative evaluation of saliency-based explainable artificial intelligence (xai) methods in deep learning-based mammogram analysis. Eur J Radiol. 2024;173:111356.
24. Muddamsetty SM, Jahromi MNS, Moeslund TB. Expert level evaluations for explainable AI (xai) methods in the medical domain. In: International conference on pattern recognition. Springer; 2021. pp. 35–46.
25. Narayanan M, Chen E, He J, Kim B, Gershman S, Doshi-Velez F. How do humans understand explanations from machine learning systems? an evaluation of the human-interpretability of explanation. arXiv preprint arXiv:1802.00682. 2018.
26. Liu C-F, Chen Z-C, Kuo S-C, Lin T-C. Does AI explainability affect physicians' intention to use AI? Int J Med Inform. 2022;168:104884.
27. Bas HM, der Velden V, Kuijf HJ, Gilhuijs KGA, Viergever MA. Explainable artificial intelligence (xai) in deep learning-based medical image analysis. Med Image Anal. 2022;79:102470.

Medical Images Analysis Through Artificial Intelligence Techniques with Explainable Features

Fulvio Bergantin, Agostino Forestiero, and Davide Macrì

Contents

Abstract The increasing prevalence of respiratory diseases, including the recent COVID-19 pandemic, underscores the need for advanced diagnostic tools that can enhance early detection and management strategies. This paper introduces a refined approach using the U-Net neural network architecture for the analysis of chest images, aimed at improving the outcomes in the diagnosis of respiratory ailments. The U-Net model, originally designed for biomedical image segmentation, is adapted here to exploit its robust feature extraction capabilities that are critical for handling the complexities associated with chest radiographs, such as variability in organ size, shape, and pathological manifestations. Through a series of transpose convolutions, pooling, and concatenation layers, the model captures intricate details across multiple spatial scales, significantly improving the accuracy of segmentation and detection tasks. This study not only explores the architecture's efficiency in segmenting and classifying these images but also enhances it with explainable AI techniques to ensure transparency and reliability in automated decision-making.

F. Bergantin · A. Forestiero · D. Macrì (✉)
Institute for High-Performance Computing and Networking, National Research Council, Rende, (CS), Italy
e-mail: fulvio.bergantin@icar.cnr.it; agostino.forestiero@icar.cnr.it; davide.macri@icar.cnr.it

R. Ortale et al. (eds.), *Explainable Machine Intelligence in Healthcare*,
https://doi.org/10.1007/978-3-031-91379-2_11

Keywords Medical images · Explainable AI · COVID-19 · U-Net architecture · Classification · Grad-CAM

1 Introduction

Medical imaging plays a vital role in diagnosing and treating various illnesses, enabling clinics to view inside structures and identify pathological conditions. Recent advances in deep learning have significantly improved medical image analysis capabilities, leading to higher diagnosis accuracy and efficacy. Among these advancements, the U-Net architecture has proven particularly effective for semantic segmentation in biomedical images, particularly for tasks requiring precise localization and identification of anatomical structures and lesions [11].

Considering the impressive capabilities of deep learning models, their application in medical imaging faces significant challenges related to interpretability and transparency. The "black-box" nature of these models frequently hinders their acceptance in clinical settings, where understanding the reasoning behind diagnostic decisions is essential to ensuring trust and dependability. The goal of artificial intelligence (XAI) is to overcome this issue by providing methods and techniques that make the decision-making processes of AI models more transparent and understandable to human experts [3].

This paper thoroughly investigates the integration of recognition technologies with a U-Net-based architecture for medical image analysis, accurately identifying COVID-19 via chest radiography [15]. The proposed approach uses a cutting-edge XAI method called Gradient-weighted Class Activation Mapping (Grad-CAM) [16] to improve the interpretability of the model's predictions. Combining the strength of U-Net [11] for accurate image segmentation with the transparency provided by XAI technology, the goal is to develop a more trustworthy and reliable diagnostic tool for clinical use.

The primary goal of this research is to create a U-Net-based framework for the segmentation and classification of chest pictures with the aim of identifying COVID-19, other respiratory illnesses (non-COVID), or a normal state devoid of disorders (normal). The following are some of the specific goals: (i) Create a custom U-Net architecture for thoracic image segmentation that can precisely identify regions of interest; (ii) Add Grad-CAM to the U-Net framework to visualize and interpret model predictions, enhancing its transparency and dependability; (iii) Test the suggested framework on a dataset that is accessible to the public in order to assess its performance in terms of explainability and segmentation accuracy.

The U-Net architecture was chosen for its effectiveness in learning from limited training data and accurately capturing fine-grained details, specifically for biomedical image segmentation. This architecture features a contracting path and an expansive path. The contracting path captures the input image's context using convolutional layers with ReLU activations and max-pooling layers for downsampling, which reduces resolution and increases the receptive field. This sequence helps us learn the spatial hierarchy and important components of the image. The expansive path reconstructs the spatial dimensions to produce the final segmented output. It includes upsampling operations, concatenation with corresponding feature maps from the contracting path, and additional convolutional layers to refine segmentation. The upsampling uses methods like transposed convolutions to enhance the feature maps' resolution. At each step, the upsampled feature maps are concatenated with the contracting path's feature maps, preserving fine-grained details lost during downsampling. This skip connection method significantly enhances the model's ability to provide precise segmentation borders, making U-Net highly effective for biomedical image analysis. The significance of this study lies in its ability to bridge the gap between the high performance of deep learning models and the requirement for interpretability in clinical settings. Providing a framework that combines the strength points of U-Net for precise image segmentation with the transparency provided by XAI technologies [6], this research aims to facilitate the use of AI-based diagnostic tools in healthcare assistance. The ability to interpret and validate the model's predictions boosts clinician confidence and ensures that AI systems may be used responsibly and ethically in critical medical applications.

This paper is organized as follows. Section 2 reviews a selection of related works; Sect. 3 describes our proposed method of analysis detailing the neural network implemented and the artificial intelligence techniques exploited; in Sect. 4 some performed tests on COVID-19 dataset were reported; and finally, Sect. 5 concludes and discusses the proposed methodology.

2 Related Works

Many studies on this topic have been proposed in the last few years. To improve the model's transparency and interpretability, a deep learning (DL)-based technique for gastrointestinal tract segmentation utilizing a 3D U-Net model was introduced in [8]. Explainable artificial intelligence (XAI) approaches are used in this approach. Automating the labor-intensive manual gastrointestinal organ outlining procedure prior to radiation therapy aims to save treatment time and labor and increase overall treatment efficiency. Using XAI techniques like GradCAM and DeepLIF, the suggested model achieves an 86.5 testing accuracy. This novel technique seeks to enable healthcare providers to treat gastrointestinal cancer patients with greater knowledge by making the organ segmentation process more transparent and understandable.

A thorough analysis of the most recent approaches to biomedical picture segmentation is given in [4]. In the first section, segmentation techniques are reviewed, and the better performance of fully convolutional neural networks (FCNN) over conventional methods is highlighted. Dilated convolution is then explored as a way to improve resolution without requiring as many pooling and downsampling layers. In order to address the "gridding" problem with dilated convolution, the paper makes reference to sequential hybrid convolutions, which are employed as solutions in

Deeplab models. Additionally, semi-dilated convolution is introduced in this study, which uses an arrangement of scalograms to increase the receptive field unevenly. The study suggests "double-dilated convolution," a sophisticated type of dilated convolution that uses two dilation variables as a way to further enhance medical image segmentation. This method's efficacy is illustrated with a publicly accessible dataset on breast cancer [1].

In [5], the segmentation of medical pictures is studied with an emphasis on lesions related to multiple sclerosis (MS). In order to overcome the difficulties associated with precise lesion localization and spatial resolution, this work incorporates attention mechanisms, which have increased segmentation models' effectiveness by sharpening focus on pertinent image regions. In order to improve the accuracy of MS lesion segmentation, the GAU-U-Net model combines Global Attention Upsample units with sophisticated convolutional neural network architecture.

Examines computer-aided medical diagnostics with a focus on pulmonary tuberculosis [14], one of the most common infectious disease-related deaths. The study tackles the problems of inaccurate diagnosis and restricted access to radiologists in communities with limited resources and remote locations. It uses deep learning algorithms for the segmentation and classification of chest radiographs in order to correctly detect tuberculosis. Radiography picture datasets of various sizes are used to train the UNet segmentation and Xception classification models. Furthermore, by employing Gradient-weighted Class Activation Mapping (Grad-CAM) to highlight anomalies associated with tuberculosis in chest X-rays, the study explores the visualization potential of these models.

In [10], kidney tumor segmentation is addressed by applying Grad-CAM. Kidney tumor segmentation is a crucial task in medical image analysis due to the often asymptomatic nature of these tumors, requiring early and precise detection for effective treatment. Recent advancements in neural networks, particularly in U-Net-based architectures, have shown significant potential in this domain. Traditional U-Net models have been highly effective for image segmentation but suffer from high computational demands, limiting their practical application in clinical settings. To address these challenges, the UNet-PWP architecture was implemented in this paper, introducing adaptive partitioning and weight pruning techniques. Adaptive partitioning breaks down the U-Net model into smaller submodels, reducing computational complexity and enhancing efficiency. Additionally, weight pruning eliminates redundant parameters, further optimizing the model without compromising accuracy. Furthermore, the integration of explainable AI techniques, such as attention mechanisms and Grad-CAM, ensures the model's decision-making process is transparent and interpretable, a crucial element for clinical trust and adoption. These innovations collectively represent a significant advancement in the practical application of deep learning for medical image segmentation.

3 Medical Image Analysis Using Explainable U-Net Architecture

This section outlines the methodology used to develop and implement a U-Net-based framework for segmenting and classifying medical images, focusing on improving interpretability and transparency through explainability techniques. The U-Net architecture was selected for its effectiveness in learning from a few training images and maintaining high accuracy in capturing fine details, particularly in biomedical image segmentation. This architecture comprises a contracting path, which captures the context of input images through convolutional and max-pooling layers, and an expansive path, which reconstructs the spatial dimensions through upsampling and concatenation with feature maps from the contracting path.

Explainable AI (XAI) techniques, particularly Gradient-weighted Class Activation Mapping (Grad-CAM), were integrated into the framework to enhance model transparency [13]. Grad-CAM helps visualize the regions of the image that the model focuses on for its predictions, thereby making the decision-making process more understandable to clinicians.

3.1 U-Net Architecture

U-Net is a widely used deep learning architecture for semantic segmentation, especially known for biomedical image analysis. It is effective on limited datasets, making it ideal for medical imaging tasks where annotated data is scarce [9].

A convolutional neural network (CNN) like U-Net consists of multiple layers trained to identify different features in an image. Each image is processed through these layers, applying various filters at different resolutions. Each layer's output serves as the next input, refining the features gradually [2]. The U-Net's U-shaped structure includes an encoder and a decoder. The encoder downscales the image to reduce spatial dimensions and capture context, using multiple stages of convolutions and pooling. The bottleneck between the encoder and decoder further processes the compressed feature maps (Fig. 1).

The decoder path upscales the feature maps to restore the image dimensions, using upsampling layers and concatenating them with corresponding encoder feature maps through skip connections. This combination preserves fine details and improves segmentation accuracy. The final output is produced after additional convolutions. Skip connections are crucial in U-Net, enabling the network to utilize high-resolution data from the encoder, enhancing segmentation precision. U-Net's ability to perform data augmentation, such as rotations and shifts, helps increase the training dataset size and model robustness, which is essential for medical imaging with limited data. U-Net's adaptability extends beyond its initial design, successfully applying to various medical imaging tasks like tumor detection and organ delineation, demonstrating its versatility.

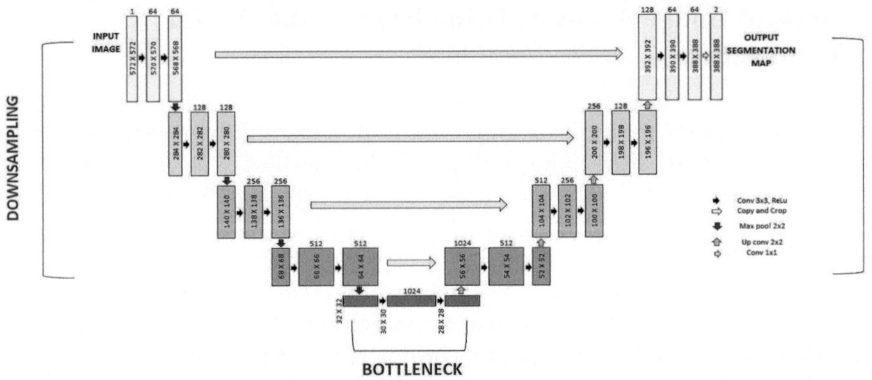

Fig. 1 Example of the U-Net architecture. Each colored box represents a multi-channel feature map. The number of channels is indicated above each box, while the spatial dimensions are specified inside the box. The arrows illustrate the various operations performed

In summary, U-Net is a powerful and flexible tool for semantic segmentation in medical imaging. Its unique encoder-decoder structure with skip connections allows it to learn complex features and provide detailed segmentations, even with limited training data, making it invaluable for researchers and medical professionals.

3.2 *Explainable AI*

Explainable artificial intelligence (XAI) is essential in today's technological environment because it makes artificial intelligence (AI) systems' decisions more transparent and understandable [12]. This idea is becoming more and more important in a variety of industries, most notably healthcare, where knowing the reasoning behind algorithmic suggestions can have a big impact on the standard of care.

The ability of XAI to offer a transparent "black box," enabling specialists to comprehend the reasoning behind AI models' decisions, is a crucial feature. In order to assess the ramifications of a diagnosis recommended by an algorithm, this transparency is essential. Medical experts are able to carefully review an image's features or any other data that went into making a certain diagnosis or recommendation. This clarity improves the decision-making process itself and helps to build trust in AI-assisted decision-making. Specialists are able to recognize biases or limitations in AI models and make the required corrections or enhancements based on their clinical expertise and understanding.

This ongoing feedback loop between AI and human operators could gradually increase the precision and effectiveness of decision support systems. Furthermore, there are moral and legal advantages to XAI. The capacity to provide an explanation for AI system actions is crucial for accountability and traceability in delicate domains such as healthcare. Concerns about privacy, security, and legal liability can be reduced by making sure that diagnosis and treatment recommendations are clear-cut and rational.

To sum up, explainable AI is a critical component of ethical AI development and use. By fostering openness, understanding, and accountability, it goes beyond being a simple technological tool and helps to create a future where AI is not only powerful and efficient but also dependable, equitable, and focused on people.

An attention visualization method called Grad-CAM (Gradient-weighted Class Activation Mapping) [16] was used to determine which areas of an image have the greatest influence on a convolutional neural network's (CNN) classification decision, specifically in a U-Net network. For a particular class of interest, Grad-CAM computes gradients with respect to the output of the neural network's last convolutional layer. Each pixel in the image's sensitivity to the target class is shown by these gradients. A class activation map is then produced by combining the gradients and weighting them according to significance. When Grad-CAM is applied to images, the regions that the model deemed important for a specific classification decision can be visualized in an understandable and straightforward manner.

Grad-CAM, for example, can be used in medical diagnostics to highlight particular image elements (such as textures or forms) that impacted the model's determination of whether a pathological state was present. Grad-CAM also makes it easier to analyze models, which helps practitioners and researchers understand the inner workings of deep learning models. It offers an open way to examine the logic underlying CNN judgments, which promotes confidence and comprehension in AI-powered applications, particularly in vital domains like healthcare.

3.3 Methodology

As part of this study's methodology, a U-Net-based framework for segmenting and classifying medical pictures is developed and implemented. Explainability techniques are also used to improve interpretability and transparency.

The U-Net architecture was chosen because it effectively learned from a few training photos and accurately captured fine-grained information. It was specifically created for biomedical image segmentation. This architecture consists of an expansive path that reconstructs the spatial dimensions to provide the final segmented output and a contracting path that uses a sequence of convolutional and max-pooling layers to capture the context of the input images. While the expansive path entails upsampling operations, concatenations with corresponding feature maps from the contracting path, and additional convolutional layers to refine the segmentation, the contracting path consists of convolutional layers with ReLU activations, followed by max-pooling layers for downsampling. The rectified linear unit (ReLU) activation function is applied after each layer of 3×3 convolutions in the contraction route, which begins with an input picture. These convolutions aid in learning the spatial hierarchy and identifying important components of the input image. Then, by employing max-pooling layers with a 2×2 window, the spatial dimensions are progressively lowered, hence increasing the receptive field and decreasing the resolution.

The model can now gather contextual information from larger areas of the image, thanks to this downsampling technique, which is essential for precise segmentation. The expanding path increases the spatial dimensions to reconstruct the image once the image representation is compressed into a bottleneck at the deepest layer of the U-Net. Upsampling methods, like transposed convolutions, are used to improve the resolution of the feature maps. The upsampled feature maps are concatenated with the corresponding feature maps from the contracting path at each step of the upsampling procedure. By preserving fine-grained information that are lost during downsampling, the skip connection method enhances the model's capacity to provide precise segmentation borders.

A flowchart that illustrates the procedure mentioned above will be included to improve understanding (Fig. 2).

Fig. 2 Flux diagram

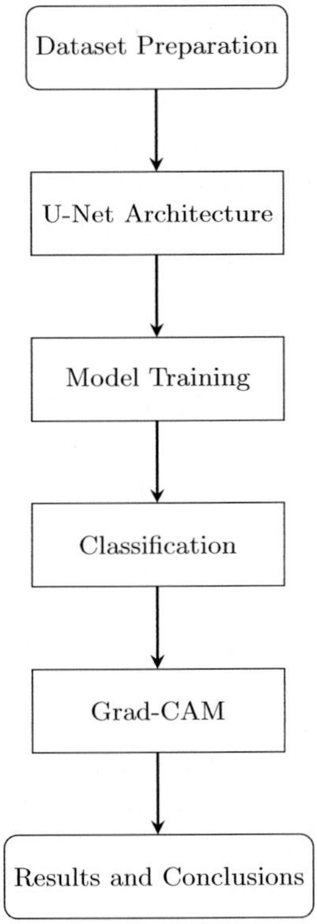

The skip connections will be highlighted in this diagram, demonstrating the concatenation of the respective upsampled feature maps with the feature maps from the contracting path. From the original input image through the several phases of downsampling and upsampling to the final segmented output, this graphic aid attempts to make the procedure more understandable. The diagram's graphical depiction will help to clarify how the model reconstructs spatial dimensions and captures context, which will enhance the segmentation process' interpretability. This inclusion highlights the study's methodological integrity and transparency.

4 Experimental Evaluation

4.1 Dataset

A dataset was evaluated using the network. This dataset is highly effective for rapidly and accurately identifying COVID-19, enabling the diagnosis of respiratory disorders using chest X-rays. The COVID-QU-Ex [15] collection consists of 33,920 chest X-ray images evenly distributed among COVID-19, non-COVID pneumonia, and normal cases. The size and diversity of this dataset significantly enhance the robustness and reliability of diagnostic models trained on it.

This dataset has demonstrated its utility in developing models that achieve high accuracy in both binary and multi-class classifications, as well as in differentiating between COVID-19 and other respiratory disorders in future diagnostic studies. The study highlights that improving the quality and generalizability of medical image classification models necessitates larger dataset sizes and the use of ensemble CNN approaches. Consequently, the COVID-QU-Ex dataset is a valuable resource for current and future research in medical diagnostics.

4.2 Performance Metrics

The performance of the proposed framework is assessed using standard evaluation metrics, including precision, recall, F-Measure, and accuracy.

Precision measures the accuracy of positive predictions made by the model. It is determined by dividing the number of true positive predictions (true positives) by the total number of positive predictions. The formula for precision is

$$\text{Precision} = \frac{\text{TP}}{\text{TP} + \text{FP}}$$

where TP represents true positives and FP stands for false positives.

Recall, also known as sensitivity, evaluates the model's ability to identify all relevant instances in the dataset correctly. It is calculated as the ratio of true positive predictions to the total number of actual positive instances. The recall formula is

$$\text{Recall} = \frac{\text{TP}}{\text{TP} + \text{FN}}$$

where FN indicates false negatives.

The F-Measure, or F1 score, is the harmonic mean of precision and recall, offering a balanced evaluation by integrating both metrics. The F-Measure is computed as

$$\text{F-Measure} = 2 \times \frac{\text{Precision} \times \text{Recall}}{\text{Precision} + \text{Recall}}$$

Accuracy indicates the proportion of correct predictions out of all predictions made by the model. It is a simple yet effective metric for assessing overall model performance. The formula for accuracy is

$$\text{Accuracy} = \frac{\text{TP} + \text{TN}}{\text{TP} + \text{TN} + \text{FP} + \text{FN}}$$

where TN denotes true negatives.

4.3 Experimental Results

The metrics reported in Sect. 4.2 were evaluated on a computational setup using an NVIDIA DGX Station with four Tesla V100 Tensor Core GPUs. To ensure the consistency and reliability of the results, a tenfold cross-validation method was utilized in all experimental evaluations.

Table 1 presents the performance metrics of the U-Net model across different classes (COVID-19, non-COVID, and normal) in terms of precision, recall, F1 score, and accuracy. The precision values indicate that the model is highly accurate in predicting true positive cases for each class, with COVID-19 achieving the highest precision at 79.41%. The recall values show the model's ability to correctly identify all relevant instances, with the highest recall observed for the normal class at 75.70%. The F1 score, which balances precision and recall, reflects the overall effectiveness of the model, demonstrating solid performance across all classes.

Table 1 Analysis of metrics

U-Net				
	Precision	Recall	F1 score	Accuracy
Covid-19	79,41	67,50	72,97	82,70
Non covid	62,50	64,10	63,29	82,70
Normal	67,43	75,70	71,26	82,70

The accuracy metric, consistently at 82.70% for all classes, highlights the model's robustness and reliability in correctly diagnosing respiratory conditions.

These results underscore the model's strong capability in differentiating between COVID-19, other respiratory illnesses, and normal cases, validating the effectiveness of the enhanced U-Net framework. This robust performance highlights the framework's potential as a reliable diagnostic tool in medical imaging, offering precise segmentation and classification. Incorporating advanced techniques, such as multi-resolution blocks and sophisticated skip connections, has significantly improved the model's accuracy and ability to capture intricate details across various scales.

The models' performance was also assessed using the confusion matrix, as shown in Fig. 3. We can pinpoint the model's achievements and shortcomings, thanks to the confusion matrix, which comprehensively comprehends the prediction outputs.

The structure is made up of rows and columns, where the rows stand for the ground truth (actual labels) and the columns stand for the labels the model predicted. Accuracy, precision, recall, F1 score, and other performance metrics are computed, errors are found using FP and FN analysis, models are optimized, and classes are assessed (i.e., which performs better) using the confusion matrix.

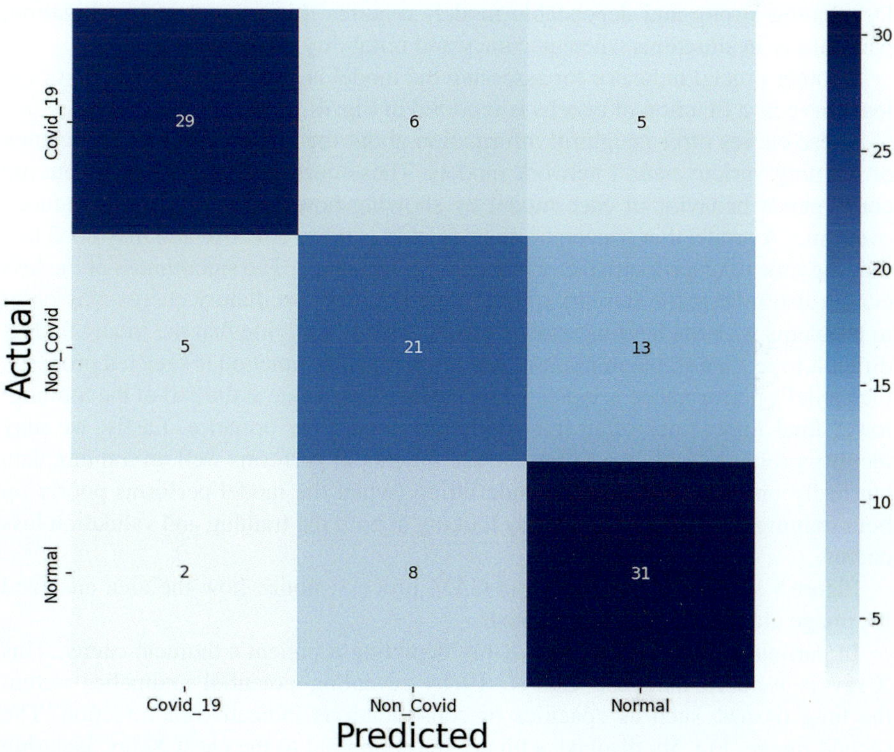

Fig. 3 Confusion matrix

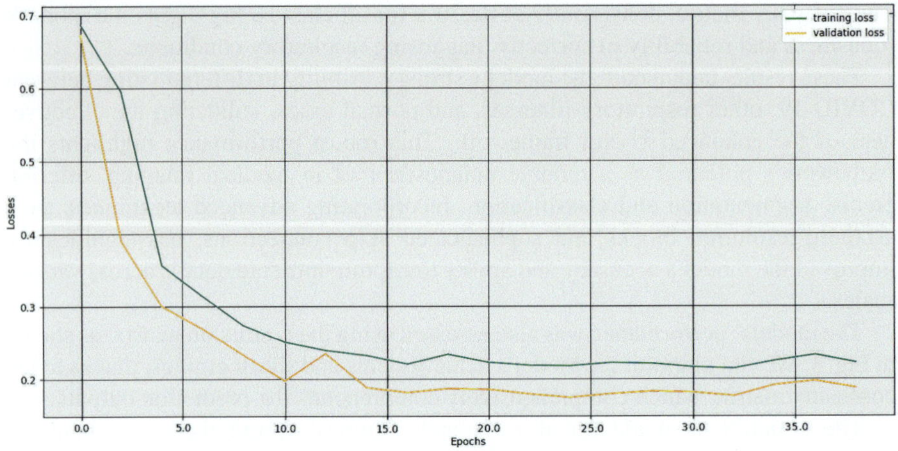

Fig. 4 Losses vs. epochs

Confusion matrices provide thorough insights on performance, mistake causes, and opportunities for development, making them an essential part of model evaluation. Developing strong and dependable models requires this amount of investigation, particularly in situations where accuracy and reliability are paramount.

Another crucial indicator for assessing the model is Losses vs. Epoch [7], or the loss curve as a function of epochs is reported in Fig. 4.

These curves offer insightful information about the effectiveness and efficiency of learning various neural network models. These curves allow us to evaluate the convergence behavior of each model by showing how rapidly its loss is reduced over time. A model that converges more quickly is more effective and may need less training time to reach a satisfactory level of performance. The smoothness of the loss curves also reveals the stability of training: extremely oscillatory curves may point to problems with the learning rate or model design, implying that the model finds it difficult to reach a stable minimum. Assuming the loss function is selected properly, the model's performance is indicated by the final loss value at the end of the training: lower final loss values often indicate higher model performance. Lastly, we may identify problems with overfitting (where the model performs well on training data but badly on validation data) or underfitting (when the model performs poorly on both training and validation data) by looking at both the training and validation loss curves.

Figure 5 visually shows the Grad-CAM process; notice how the area analyzed for image classification is highlighted.

In particular, Fig. 5a is a chest X-ray depicting a patient's thoracic cavity. This X-ray is used to diagnose COVID-19 by revealing potential anomalies within the lung tissues, such as opacities or consolidations indicative of infection. The second image, Fig. 5b, displays a binary mask applied to the chest X-ray, isolating the lung regions. The white areas represent the segmented lungs, which are

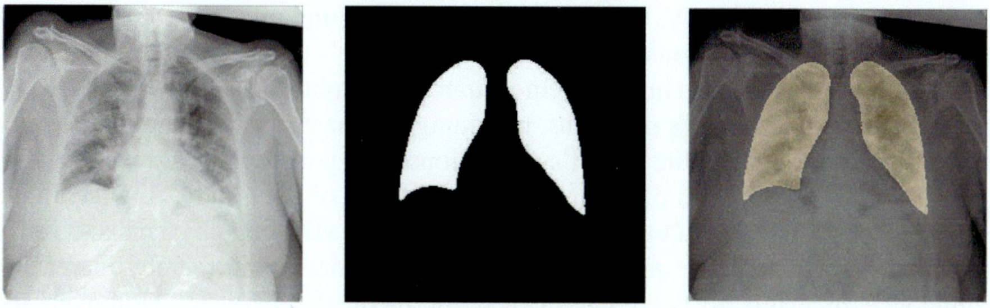

(a) (b) (c)

Fig. 5 A sample image of COVID-19 dataset with its mask and Grad-CAM explainability. (**a**) Sample image. (**b**) Sample image mask. (**c**) Grad-CAM explainability

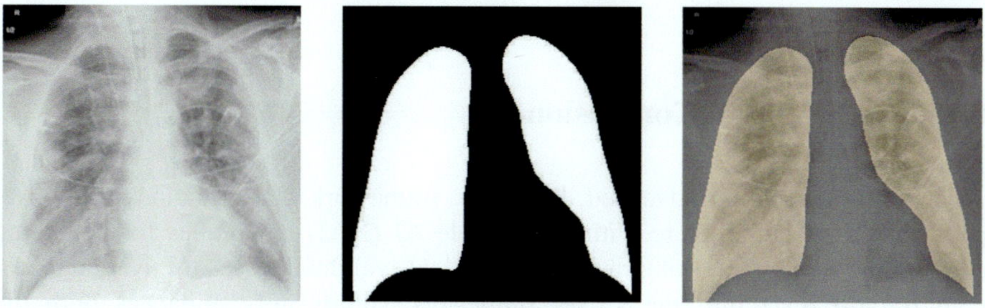

(a) (b) (c)

Fig. 6 A second sample image of COVID-19 dataset with its mask and Grad-CAM explainability. (**a**) Sample image 2. (**b**) Sample image mask 2. (**c**) Grad-CAM explainability

essential for focused image processing and analysis to improve the accuracy of detecting lung-related pathologies. The third image, Fig. 5c, shows a Grad-CAM (Gradient-weighted Class Activation Mapping) overlay on the chest X-ray. This visualization technique highlights the specific regions of the lungs that the AI model emphasizes when making its predictions, thereby providing insights into the model's interpretability and decision-making process.

After analyzing an example of the Grad-CAM application on a chest X-ray for COVID-19 diagnosis, it is beneficial to examine another use case to better understand the versatility and effectiveness of this technique. The second example shown in Fig. 6 also confirms that the Grad-CAM explainability technique is reliable and repeatable across all images in the analyzed dataset.

Specifically, Fig. 6a represents a chest X-ray, but this time, it is used to identify another pulmonary pathology, such as pneumonia. The chest X-ray is examined to detect anomalies in the lung tissues, such as inflammations or consolidations indicative of lung infections. The second image, Fig. 6b, displays a binary mask applied to the X-ray, isolating the lung regions for a more detailed analysis. The white areas indicate the segmented lungs, which are essential for improving the accuracy of lung pathology detection. The last image, Fig. 6c, presents a Grad-CAM overlay on the chest X-ray, highlighting the specific lung areas that the AI model focuses on for its predictions.

This second example further demonstrates the robustness of Grad-CAM in interpreting the AI model's decisions, providing a clear visualization of the regions of interest that influence the model's predictions. The consistency of results across different chest X-ray examples reinforces the validity of the Grad-CAM technique as a valuable tool for explainability in clinical contexts, allowing physicians to verify and better understand the decisions made by neural networks, thereby increasing confidence in using artificial intelligence for medical diagnosis. Moreover, the ability to visualize and interpret AI-driven decisions is crucial for regulatory compliance and accepting AI systems in clinical practice. This not only aids in identifying potential errors but also supports ongoing improvements in AI models, ensuring they remain effective and trustworthy tools in medical diagnostics.

5 Discussion and Conclusions

This study presents an advanced diagnostic framework that combines the U-Net neural network architecture with explainable AI (XAI) techniques for analyzing chest radiographs. The integration of Gradient-weighted Class Activation Mapping (Grad-CAM) into the U-Net framework significantly enhances both the segmentation and classification accuracy while improving the transparency and interpretability of the model's decisions. The results, evaluated on the COVID-QU-Ex dataset, demonstrate the robustness of our approach, achieving high precision, recall, F1 score, and accuracy in distinguishing between COVID-19, other respiratory illnesses, and normal cases.

The U-Net architecture, renowned for its encoder-decoder structure and skip connections, has proven highly effective for biomedical image segmentation. Its capability to capture intricate details across multiple spatial scales is essential for managing the complexities of chest radiographs. By incorporating Grad-CAM, our framework addresses the critical need for transparency in AI-driven diagnostics. This inclusion allows for the visualization and interpretation of model predictions, which fosters trust among clinicians and enhances the acceptance of AI tools in clinical settings.

The performance metrics indicate that our model performs reliably across different classes. High scores in these metrics reflect the model's efficacy in accurately diagnosing respiratory conditions, which is vital for clinical applications. The use of the COVID-QU-Ex dataset, a comprehensive collection of chest X-ray images, provided a robust testbed for our framework. The tenfold cross-validation method ensured the reliability and generalizability of the results, highlighting the potential of our approach in real-world clinical scenarios. Furthermore, while the study focused on COVID-19 detection, the adaptability of the U-Net architecture suggests that our framework can be extended to other medical imaging tasks. This ability to generalize across different datasets and medical conditions makes it a versatile tool in the broader context of medical diagnostics.

Nevertheless, it is essential to acknowledge the limitations and areas for future improvement. Although the COVID-QU-Ex dataset is extensive, further validation on more diverse datasets would enhance the generalizability of our approach. Additionally, the reliance on high-performance computing resources may limit the accessibility of this approach in resource-constrained settings. Future work could focus on optimizing the model for deployment on less powerful hardware.

In conclusion, the combination of U-Net and XAI techniques offers a powerful and interpretable framework for medical image analysis. The promising results and enhanced transparency make it a valuable tool for clinicians, paving the way for more trustworthy and reliable AI-driven diagnostics in healthcare.

References

1. Al-Dhabyani W, Gomaa M, Khaled H, Fahmy A. Dataset of breast ultrasound images. Data Brief. 2020;28:104863.
2. Bodapati JD, Sajja R, Naralasetti V. An efficient approach for semantic segmentation of salt domes in seismic images using improved unet architecture. J Inst Eng (India): Series B. 2023;104(3):569–78.
3. Doshi-Velez F, Kim B. Towards a rigorous science of interpretable machine learning. arXiv: Machine Learning. 2017.
4. Farrag A, Gad G, Fadlullah ZM, Fouda MM, Alsabaan M. An explainable AI system for medical image segmentation with preserved local resolution: Mammogram tumor segmentation. IEEE Access. 2023.
5. Gamal R, Barka H, Hadhoud M. Gau u-net for multiple sclerosis segmentation. Alex Eng J. 2023;73:625–34.
6. Hulsen T. Explainable artificial intelligence (xai): Concepts and challenges in healthcare. AI. 2023;4(3):652–66.
7. Ishida T, Yamane I, Sakai T, Niu G, Sugiyama M. Do we need zero training loss after achieving zero training error? arXiv preprint arXiv:2002.08709. 2020.
8. Kai Li, Chan J. Gastro-intestinal tract segmentation using an explainable 3D unet. arXiv preprint arXiv:2309.14474. 2023.
9. Morani K, Ayana EK, Kollias D, Unay D. Detecting covid-19 in computed tomography images: A novel approach utilizing segmentation with unet architecture, lung extraction, and cnn classifier. In: Science and information conference. Springer; 2024. pp. 450–65.
10. Rao PK, Chatterjee S, Janardhan M, Nagaraju K, Khan SB, Almusharraf A, Alharbe AI. Optimizing inference distribution for efficient kidney tumor segmentation using a unet-pwp deep-learning model with xai on ct scan images. Diagnostics. 2023;13(20):3244.
11. Ronneberger O, Fischer P, Brox T. U-net: Convolutional networks for biomedical image segmentation. In: Lecture notes in computer science. 2015. pp. 234–41.
12. Saeed W, Omlin C. Explainable AI (XAI): A systematic meta-survey of current challenges and future opportunities. ArXiv. abs/2111.06420. 2021.
13. Selvaraju RR, Das A, Vedantam R, Cogswell M, Parikh D, Batra D. Grad-cam: Visual explanations from deep networks via gradient-based localization. Int J Comput Vis. 2016;128:336–59.
14. Sharma V, Gupta SK, Shukla KK, et al. Deep learning models for tuberculosis detection and infected region visualization in chest x-ray images. Intell Med. 2023.

15. Tahir AM, Muhammad E, Chowdhury H, Qiblawey Y, Khandakar A, Rahman T, Kiranyaz S, Khurshid U, Ibtehaz N, Mahmud S, Ezeddin M. Covid-qu-ex dataset. 2022.
16. Wang Z, Zhang T, Huang X. Explainable deep learning for image-driven fire calorimetry. Appl Intell. 2024;54(1):1047–62.

MIX
Papier aus verantwortungsvollen Quellen
Paper from responsible sources
FSC® C105338

If you have any concerns about our products,
you can contact us on
ProductSafety@springernature.com

In case Publisher is established outside the EU,
the EU authorized representative is:
Springer Nature Customer Service Center GmbH
Europaplatz 3, 69115 Heidelberg, Germany

Printed by Libri Plureos GmbH
in Hamburg, Germany